BenBella Books, Inc.

SOUL HEALING MIRACLES

"Dr. Sha makes available secret techniques and insights that were available in the past only to a select few. He shares in simple terms the insights and tools that took him more than thirty years of hard work and discipline to attain. He gives you access to information that would otherwise be unattainable."

—Dr. John Gray,
author of *Men Are from Mars, Women Are from Venus*

"We, the human race, need more Zhi Gang Sha."

—Dr. Maya Angelou,
author of *I Know Why the Caged Bird Sings*

"Dr. Sha offers a clear, practical path to learning the secrets of self-healing."

—Marianne Williamson,
author of *A Return to Love*

"Practical, useful information and techniques for putting the body's natural abilities to work on healing—a wonderful contribution."

—Dr. Wayne Dyer,
author of *There's a Spiritual Solution to Every Problem*

"Dr. Sha is an important teacher and a wonderful healer with a valuable message about the power of the soul to influence and transform all life."

—Dr. Masaru Emoto,
author of *The Hidden Messages in Water*

Soul Healing Miracles

Ancient and New Sacred Wisdom, Knowledge, and Practical Techniques for Healing the Spiritual, Mental, Emotional, and Physical Bodies

DR. AND MASTER
Zhi Gang Sha

BENBELLA BOOKS, INC.

DALLAS, TEXAS

BenBella Books, Inc.
10300 N. Central Expressway
Suite #530
Dallas, TX 75231
www.benbellabooks.com
Send feedback to feedback@benbellabooks.com

Heaven's Library and Soul Healing Miracles Series are trademarks
of Heaven's Library Publication Corp.
First hardcover edition November 2013

Printed in the United States of America
10 9 8 7 6 5 4 3 2

Library of Congress Cataloging-in-Publication Data is available for this title upon request.
ISBN: 978-1-940363-07-3

Text design and composition by John Reinhardt Book Design
Proofreading by Michael Fedison and Kimberly Marini
Indexing by Clive Pyne Book Indexing Services
Printed by Bang Printing

Distributed by Perseus Distribution
www.perseusdistribution.com

To place orders through Perseus Distribution:
Tel: (800) 343-4499
Fax: (800) 351-5073
E-mail: orderentry@perseusbooks.com

Significant discounts for bulk sales are available.
Please contact Glenn Yeffeth at glenn@benbellabooks.com or (214) 750-3628.

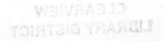

Contents

Foreword to the Soul Healing Miracles Series

I HAVE ADMIRED DR. ZHI GANG SHA'S WORK for some years now. In fact, I clearly remember the first time I heard him describe his soul healing system of Soul Mind Body Medicine. I immediately knew that I wanted to support this gifted healer and his mission, so I introduced him to my spiritual community. Ever since, it has been my joy to witness how those who apply his teachings and techniques experience increased energy, joy, harmony, and peace in their lives.

Dr. Sha's techniques awaken the healing power already present in all sentient beings, empowering them by placing their well-being directly in their own hands. His explanation of how energy and message link consciousness, mind, body, and spirit forms a dynamic information network in language that is easy to understand and, more important, to apply.

Dr. Sha's time-tested results have proved to thousands of students and readers that healing energies and messages exist within specific sounds, movements, and perceptions. Sharing and demonstrating this in his own personal life, Dr. Sha's theories and practices of working with the life force are holistic, profound, and practical. His message that Soul Power is applicable to every aspect of life makes it possible for aspiring practitioners to have confidence that they can successfully navigate the challenges of twenty-first-century living.

As the worldwide representative of his renowned teacher, Dr. Zhi Chen Guo, who was one of the greatest qi gong masters and healers in the world, Dr. Sha is himself a master of ancient disciplines, including tai chi, qi gong, kung fu, *I Ching*, and feng shui. He has succeeded in blending the soul of his culture's natural healing methods with his training as a Western physician, generously offering his wisdom to us through the books of his Soul Power Series and Soul Healing Miracles Series.

Dr. Sha's contribution to those in the healing community is undeniable, and the way in which he empowers his readers to understand themselves, their feelings, emotions, and the interconnection of their body, mind, and spirit is his gift to the evolutionary progress of the world. But that's not all. Through his books, Dr. Sha gently guides the reader into a consciousness of healing not only body, mind, and spirit, but also the heart. Through his new Soul Healing Miracles Series, Dr. Sha further empowers readers to heal their mind, body, and spirit by revealing powerful new methods of healing.

I consider Dr. Sha's healing path to be a universal spiritual practice, a journey into genuine transformation. His professional integrity and compassionate heart are at the root of his being a servant of humankind, and my heartfelt prayer for his readers is that they accept his invitation to awaken the power within their souls and realize the natural beauty of their existence.

Michael Bernard Beckwith
Author of *Life Visioning* and *Spiritual Liberation*
Founder of Agape International Spiritual Center
August 2013

Introduction to the
Soul Healing Miracles Series

I HAVE SHARED THE PURPOSE of my life in my Soul Power Series. I will emphasize further the purpose of my life in the Soul Healing Miracles Series.

The purpose of life is to serve. I have committed my life to this purpose. Service is my life mission. To serve is to make others happier and healthier.

My total life mission is to transform the soul, heart, mind, and body of humanity and all souls in Heaven, Mother Earth, and countless planets, stars, galaxies, and universes, and enlighten them or enlighten them further, in order to create the Love Peace Harmony Universal Family.

This Universal Family includes all humanity on Mother Earth and all souls in Mother Earth, Heaven, and countless planets, stars, galaxies, and universes. The ultimate goal of the Universal Family is to reach *wan ling rong he,* which is universal Oneness.

"Wan" means *ten thousand.* In Chinese "wan" represents *all.* "Ling" means *soul.* "Rong he" means *join as one.* "Wan ling rong he" (pronounced *wahn ling rawng huh*) means *all souls join as one.* This is universal Oneness. This is the ultimate goal in this new universal era. This new era, called the Soul Light Era, started on August 8, 2003 and will last fifteen thousand years.

My total life mission includes three empowerments.

My first empowerment is to teach *universal service* to empower people to be unconditional universal servants. The message of universal service is:

I serve humanity and all souls in Mother Earth, Heaven,
and countless planets, stars, galaxies, and universes unconditionally.

You serve humanity and all souls in Mother Earth, Heaven,
and countless planets, stars, galaxies, and universes unconditionally.

Together we serve humanity and all souls in Mother Earth, Heaven,
and countless planets, stars, galaxies, and universes unconditionally.

My second empowerment is to teach *soul secrets, wisdom, knowledge, and practical techniques* to empower people to create soul healing miracles to transform all life. The message is:

I have the power to create soul healing miracles
to transform all of my life.

You have the power to create soul healing miracles
to transform all of your life.

Together we have the power to create soul healing miracles
to transform all life of humanity and all souls in Mother Earth
and countless planets, stars, galaxies, and universes.

To transform all life is to:

- boost energy, stamina, vitality, and immunity
- heal the spiritual, mental, emotional, and physical bodies
- prevent all sickness
- transform all kinds of relationships
- transform finances and business
- rejuvenate soul, heart, mind, and body
- increase soul, heart, and mind intelligence
- open spiritual channels
- bring success to every aspect of life
- and more

My third empowerment is to teach *Tao* to empower people to reach Tao. To reach Tao is to reach soul mind body enlightenment.
Tao is the Source.

The Source is the Creator of Heaven, Mother Earth, and countless planets, stars, galaxies, and universes.

Tao is The Way of all life.

Tao is the universal principles and laws.

Soul enlightenment is to uplift one's soul standing in Heaven to a saint's level. The first step in the spiritual journey is to reach soul enlightenment.

A human being has two lives: physical life and soul life. Physical life is limited. Soul life is eternal. The purpose of physical life is to serve the soul life. The purpose of the soul life is to reach soul enlightenment. To reach soul enlightenment is to uplift your soul standing in Heaven in order to become a saint. To become a saint is to become a better servant. The highest saints will be uplifted to the divine realm. If one's soul reaches the divine realm, this soul has reached very high soul enlightenment.

The second step in the spiritual journey is to reach mind enlightenment.

Mind enlightenment is to uplift one's consciousness to the consciousness of a saint. The saints reside in different layers of Heaven. The consciousness of the highest saints could be uplifted further and completely transform to divine consciousness. To reach divine consciousness is beyond comprehension.

The third step in the spiritual journey is to reach body enlightenment.

Body enlightenment is to transform the physical body to the purest light body. To attain the purest light body is to reach immortality.

Let me explain the essence of immortality.

Lao Zi, the author of *Dao De Jing*, stated:

Ren Fa Di, Di Fa Tian, Tian Fa Tao, Tao Fa Zi Ran.

These four sacred phrases have explained the process of body enlightenment, which is the process of reaching immortality.

Ren Fa Di—"Ren" means *human being*. "Fa" means *follow the principles and laws*. "Di" means *Mother Earth*. "Ren Fa Di" (pronounced *wren fah dee*) means *a human being must follow the principles and laws of Mother Earth*. The law of gravity is one example.

Ren Fa Di has a deeper meaning. It teaches to transform the jing qi shen (pronounced *jing chee shun*) of a human being to the jing qi shen of Mother Earth.

"Jing" means *matter*. "Qi" means *energy*. "Shen" means *soul* or *spirit* or *message* or *information*.

One of the most important ancient secret wisdoms about universal formation can be summarized in one sentence:

Heaven, Mother Earth, human beings, and countless planets, stars, galaxies, and universes are made of jing qi shen.

Another one-sentence secret of ancient wisdom is:

Tian Ren He Yi

"Tian" means *Heaven* or *the bigger universe*. "Ren" means *human being* or *the smaller universe*. "He Yi" means *join as one*.

"Tian Ren He Yi" (pronounced *tyen wren huh yee*) means *the bigger universe and the smaller universe are one*. What the big universe has, the small universe also has, and vice versa. It teaches us the secret wisdom:

In order to understand the big universe, which includes Heaven, Mother Earth, and countless planets, stars, galaxies, and universes, understand the small universe first, which is the human being.

Lao Zi teaches us that Ren Fa Di carries the sacred meaning of transforming jing qi shen. We need to understand that the jing qi shen of a human being is *far* from the jing qi shen of Mother Earth. A human being has a potential life span of one hundred years or more. Humanity's genes could allow a human being to live to the age of 140 or 150.

How many years has Mother Earth existed? Nobody knows. At this moment, I am communicating with The Source. I am asking how long Mother Earth has lived. The answer is:

Mother Earth has lived billions of years or more.

This answer was received through my soul communication with The Source. The Source created Mother Earth. On Mother Earth the oldest minerals analyzed to date were found in Western Australia and are at least 4.4 billion years old. In the future, additional scientific study could discover even older things on Mother Earth.

Ren Fa Di teaches us very important secrets to prolong a human being's life. We have to transform the jing qi shen of a human being to the jing qi shen of Mother Earth. Therefore, in ancient teaching there is another sacred phrase:

Xi shou tian di jing hua

"Xi shou" means *absorb*. "Tian" means *Heaven*. "Di" means *Mother Earth*. "Jing hua" means *essence*. The essence is the jing qi shen of Heaven and Mother Earth. "Xi shou tian di jing hua" (pronounced *shee sho tyen dee jing hwah*) means *absorb the essence of Heaven and Mother Earth*.

Di Fa Tian—"Di" means *Mother Earth*. "Fa" means *follow the principles and laws*. "Tian" means *Heaven*. "Di Fa Tian" (pronounced *dee fah tyen*) means *Mother Earth must follow the principles and laws of Heaven*.

For longevity and to reach immortality one must first transform the jing qi shen of a human being to the jing qi shen of Mother Earth, and then further transform the jing qi shen of Mother Earth to the jing qi shen of Heaven.

Tian Fa Tao—"Tian" means *Heaven*. "Fa" means *follow the principles and laws*. "Tao" is *the Source, The Way, and the universal principles and laws*. "Tian Fa Tao" (pronounced *tyen fah dow*) means *Heaven must follow the principles and laws of Tao*.

For longevity and to reach immortality the process is:

- **Step 1:** Transform the jing qi shen of a human being to the jing qi shen of Mother Earth.
- **Step 2:** Further transform the jing qi shen of Mother Earth to the jing qi shen of Heaven.
- **Step 3:** Even further transform the jing qi shen of Heaven to the jing qi shen of Tao.
- **Step 4:** Reach Tao Fa Zi Ran (reach and meld with Tao).

Tao Fa Zi Ran—"Tao" is *the Source, The Way, and the universal principles and laws.* "Fa" means *follow the principles and laws.* "Zi Ran" means *nature.* "Tao Fa Zi Ran" (pronounced *dow fah dz rahn*) means *follow nature's way.*

To reach Tao Fa Zi Ran is to reach Tao. To reach Tao is to *meld with Tao.* To meld with Tao is to reach immortality. This is body enlightenment.

I emphasize again that my third empowerment is to empower serious spiritual seekers to reach Tao, which is to reach soul mind body enlightenment.

This is the sacred way to reach immortality.

The message of the third empowerment is:

I have the power to reach soul mind body enlightenment.

You have the power to reach soul mind body enlightenment.

Together we have the power to reach soul mind body enlightenment.

In my Soul Power Series I have shared my personal story of how the Divine chose me as a servant of humanity and the Divine in July 2003. I will not repeat the story here. Please read the books of my Soul Power Series.

As a divine servant, vehicle, and channel I have offered Divine Karma Cleansing and Divine Soul Mind Body Transplants for the last ten years. Hundreds of thousands of soul healing miracles have been created by these divine services and by thousands of soul healers that I have created on Mother Earth. Now soul healing miracles are being created every day. Therefore, the Divine and The Source guided me that the time is ready to create and write the Soul Healing Miracles Series.

I would like every reader to know that the Soul Healing Miracles Series teaches and empowers you and humanity to create your own soul healing miracles. Readers will learn sacred wisdom and knowledge and apply the practical techniques of soul healing. Everyone could create soul healing miracles.

In 2008 Tao, which is the Source, chose me as a servant of humanity and Tao. I started to offer Tao Karma Cleansing and Tao Soul Mind Body Transplants. My soul standing has been uplifted continuously over the last ten years. I am extremely honored that I have received soul uplift-ment to higher and higher layers of Source. Source has unlimited layers. Upliftment never ends. To be uplifted higher and higher is to be a better servant for humanity and all souls.

Now it is 2013. In the last ten years there have been many natural disasters in the world, including earthquakes, tsunamis, hurricanes, floods, fires, volcanic eruptions, droughts, and more. There are many other challenges, including political challenges, economic, financial and business challenges, environmental challenges, healthcare challen-ges, religious and ethnic wars, and many other challenges.

Millions of people are suffering from sickness in the spiritual body, mental body, emotional body, and physical body. Millions and millions of people worldwide have limited or no access to adequate healthcare.

Why are Mother Earth and humanity facing challenges? The reason is soul mind body blockages.

Soul blockages are bad karma. Bad karma is carried by one's soul for one's mistakes of hurting, harming, or taking advantage of others in all of one's lifetimes.

Mind blockages include negative mind-sets, negative beliefs, nega-tive attitudes, ego, attachments, and more.

Body blockages include energy blockages and matter blockages.

How to help humanity pass through this difficult historical per-iod? How to help humanity remove sickness? How to help humanity heal sickness faster? Most important: How to help humanity *prevent* sickness?

My previous books, including *Soul Mind Body Medicine*, *Power Healing*, and the ten books in my Soul Power Series, including *Soul Wisdom*, *The Power of Soul*, *Divine Soul Mind Body Healing and Transmission System*,

Tao I, and *Tao Song and Tao Dance*, have offered answers to the above "how to help humanity" questions and created hundreds of thousands of soul healing miracles worldwide.

In this new Soul Healing Miracles Series I will offer further soul secrets, wisdom, knowledge, and practical soul techniques. The teaching and practices will become simpler, more practical, more powerful, and bring soul healing miracles faster.

What are the new secrets and power that I will give you in this series? I will create The Source Field within this book. What is The Source Field? The Source Field is a field with the jing qi shen of The Source.

How does The Source Field work? The Source Field carries The Source jing qi shen with the frequency and vibration of The Source love, forgiveness, compassion, and light that can transform the jing qi shen of all unhealthy conditions.

One of the most important principles and laws in countless planets, stars, galaxies, and universes can be summarized in one sentence:

Everyone and everything in Heaven, Mother Earth, and countless planets, stars, galaxies, and universes is vibration, which is the field of jing qi shen.

The Source Field carries the jing qi shen of The Source that can remove soul mind body blockages of sickness and transform the jing qi shen of a human being's spiritual, mental, emotional, and physical bodies from head to toe, skin to bone, to restore them to health.

I will create The Source Field by writing several The Source Ling Guang Calligraphies for this book. "Ling Guang" (pronounced *ling gwahng*) means *soul light*. *The Source Ling Guang Calligraphy* is the name The Source gave to me. It means *The Source Soul Light Calligraphy*.

I will create The Source Field within each of The Source Ling Guang Calligraphies. Each one will carry the jing qi shen of The Source, which can heal and create soul healing miracles. How do these calligraphies work? The Source Ling Guang Calligraphies receive permanent treasures from The Source, which carry The Source jing qi shen. The Source jing is The Source *matter*. The Source qi is The Source *energy*. The Source shen is The Source *soul* or *message*. The Source jing qi shen field carries

The Source frequency and vibration with The Source love, forgiveness, compassion, and light that can remove soul mind body blockages of sickness for healing, rejuvenation, and creating soul healing miracles.

This is the first time that I have shared The Source Ling Guang Calligraphies with humanity. The Source Ling Guang Calligraphies can create soul healing miracles. The Source Ling Guang Calligraphies in this book are:

- The Source Ling Guang Calligraphy *Tao Guang Zha Shan* (Tao Light Explodes and Vibrates, pronounced *dow gwahng jah shahn*)
- The Source Ling Guang Calligraphy *Hei Heng Hong Ha* (The Source Zhong Mantra, pronounced *hay hung hawng hah*)
- The Source Ling Guang Calligraphy *Guang Liang Hao Mei* (Transparent Light Brings Inner and Outer Beauty, pronounced *gwahng lyahng how may*)
- The Source Ling Guang Calligraphy *Ling Guang* (Soul Light, pronounced *ling gwahng*)
- The Source Ling Guang Calligraphy *Da Ai* (Greatest Love, pronounced *dah eye*) that can melt all blockages and transform all life
- The Source Ling Guang Calligraphy *Da Kuan Shu* (Greatest Forgiveness, pronounced *dah kwahn shoo*) that can bring inner joy and inner peace to all life
- The Source Ling Guang Calligraphy *Da Ci Bei* (Greatest Compassion, pronounced *dah sz bay*) that can boost energy, stamina, vitality, and immunity of all life
- The Source Ling Guang Calligraphy *Da Guang Ming* (Greatest Light, pronounced *dah gwahng ming*) that can heal; prevent all sickness; purify and rejuvenate soul, heart, mind, and body; transform all relationships; transform business and finances; increase intelligence; open spiritual channels; and bring success to all life
- The Source Ling Guang Calligraphy *San Jiao Chang Tong* (The Key Pathway of Qi and Body Fluid Flows Freely, pronounced *sahn jee-yow chahng tawng*) that can remove soul mind body blockages of the key pathway of qi and body fluid for healing

and rejuvenation. "San" means *three*. "Jiao" means *area*. "San Jiao" (pronounced *sahn jee-yow*) is the key pathway of qi and body fluid for a person. San Jiao is the concept, wisdom, and practice of five-thousand-year-old traditional Chinese medicine. You will learn much more about the San Jiao in this book.

How can I create The Source Field in The Source Ling Guang Calligraphies? I am the servant, vehicle, and channel of The Source. The Source has given me the honor and authority to connect with The Source in order to create The Source Field.

The Source Ling Guang Calligraphies carry power beyond comprehension. Try it. Practice with it. Apply it to heal your spiritual, mental, emotional, and physical bodies. Experience the power of The Source Ling Guang Calligraphies within this book.

There are three ways to use The Source Ling Guang Calligraphies in this book:

1. Put one palm on a photograph (see list of figures on page li) of The Source Ling Guang Calligraphy. Put your other palm on any part of the body that needs healing and sincerely ask for healing.
2. Put The Source Ling Guang Calligraphy on any part of the body that needs healing. Sincerely ask for healing.
3. Meditate with The Source Ling Guang Calligraphy. Sincerely ask for healing.

There is a renowned phrase in ancient sacred spiritual teaching:

Da Tao zhi jian

"Da" means *big*. "Tao" is *The Way*. "Zhi" means *extremely*. "Jian" means *simple*. "Da Tao zhi jian" (pronounced *dah dow jr jyen*) means *The Big Way is extremely simple*. The Soul Healing Miracles Series will follow this principle. You could realize the simplicity very quickly. You could receive soul healing miracles very quickly and wonder *how?* and *why?*

I am excited, honored, and humbled to create and write this new Soul Healing Miracles Series for humanity. I cannot thank The Source, the Divine, and all Heaven's Committees enough for their sacred wisdom, knowledge, and practical techniques, as well as for their immeasurable power to bless us. How blessed humanity is that The Source puts The Source power in the books and offers permanent downloads to my readers. I am simply a servant and vessel for my readers, humanity, and all souls.

The message of soul healing miracles is:

I have the power to create soul healing miracles
to transform all of my life.

You have the power to create soul healing miracles
to transform all of your life.

Together we have the power to create soul healing miracles
to transform all life of humanity and all souls in Mother Earth
and countless planets, stars, galaxies, and universes.

I love my heart and soul
I love all humanity
Join hearts and souls together
Love, peace and harmony
Love, peace and harmony

Love all humanity. Love all souls.
Thank all humanity. Thank all souls.
Love you. Love you. Love you.
Thank you. Thank you. Thank you.

Introduction to
Soul Healing Miracles

TWENTY YEARS AGO, I joined a group of Chinese Cultural Representatives from seven provinces to visit Canada for Chinese cultural exhibitions. From watching the news, Dr. and Master Zhi Gang Sha heard about this visit and learned that I was the Cultural Representative from Shandong province. He came to visit me at my hotel in Toronto. During our meeting, I realized that he is a unique person who is very forthright and sincere, innocent, joyful, positive, extremely intelligent, and much more. His speech was amazingly refined and his responses were very quick and clear. Our meeting was very pleasant and I thoroughly enjoyed my conversation with him. Before our initial meeting ended, Dr. and Master Sha asked me if he could be my disciple to learn *I Ching* from me.

I could see that Dr. and Master Sha had already mastered his learning of traditional Chinese medicine, acupuncture, and various ancient Asian arts from many renowned masters in those areas. Therefore, I happily accepted his request to be my disciple.

During my brief stay in Canada, I taught him the essence of some aspects of *I Ching*, such as the importance of the changes of Tao in *I Ching*, including learning the balance of softness and strength, small details and broader visions, roundness and square, action and knowledge, etc.

During my private lecture with Dr. and Master Sha, I was very impressed with his extraordinary intelligence. I realized the incredible depth and breadth of his wisdom and knowledge from his responses and understanding of my teaching. With some extremely sophisticated questions such as *Why is "Yi" the source of Big Tao/The Big Way* and *Why are purity, quietness, and refined matter the essence of "Yi?"*, Dr. and

Master Sha shared with me many exceptional insights. I was extremely impressed and happy to have such an outstanding disciple!

We have stayed in close contact since we first met twenty years ago. A couple of years after my first meeting with Dr. and Master Sha, I visited him in Canada again. By then, he was already a very famous acupuncturist with a great reputation for creating abundant healing miracles in Canada. To express how proud I was of him, I gifted him my calligraphy entitled 沙氏神針 福澤億民, "Sha Shi Shen Zhen Fu Ze Yi Min" (pronounced *shah shr shun jun foo zuh yee meen*), which means *Sha's divine acupuncture, heal and benefit hundreds of millions of people*, to praise his incredible knowledge and skills of acupuncture and traditional Chinese medicine. Around that time, Dr. and Master Sha introduced Mrs. Sylvia Chen to me and recommended her to be my disciple. I happily accepted her as my disciple as well.

Because of his incredible sincerity (誠 or "cheng," pronounced *chung*) and honesty, Dr. and Master Sha has since become the founder and grandmaster of Soul Mind Body Medicine. Ancient wisdom teaches us, "Sincerity is The Way to Heaven. To think sincerely and honestly is The Way of men." Our wise forefathers thus brought sincerity and honesty into the realm of Heaven's Way (Tao). This is because sincerity and honesty have energy. Ancient Chinese wisdom says, 精誠所至, 金石為 開 "Jing cheng suo zhi, jin shi wei kai" (pronounced *jing chung swaw jr, jeen shr way kye*). This means *true sincerity and honesty can move Heaven and Earth; sincerity and honesty even have power to split metal and stone open.* In other words, if one has true sincerity and honesty, one can achieve anything in life. In *Zhong Yong, the Doctrine of the Mean* (here "mean" means *middle*), one of the ancient authoritative books on Confucianism, is written, "The Way (Tao) of ultimate sincerity and honesty enables one to foresee and understand everything."

In 2010 Zhi Gang came to China to visit his family during Chinese New Year. He and Mrs. Sylvia Chen visited me in Jinan city during that time. Mrs. Chen shared with me many stories about incredible healing miracles that Zhi Gang had created worldwide. I was extremely impressed by these healing miracles. She also brought several of his Soul Song CDs for me. When I listened to his incredibly powerful and magnificent voice, I noticed his singing created a very unique field surrounding me, which I had never experienced before. This brought me back to the pleasant experiences of my childhood. I used to dance while listening to the music I loved. Singing together with Zhi Gang brought so much profound joy to my body, heart, and mind. To express my appreciation to him and this profound experience, I wrote this couplet to praise him:

聞玄天妙音

Wen xuan tian miao yin

(pronounced *wun shwen tyen mee-yow yeen*)

Listening to the profound heavenly utterances and singing

得大道至簡

De Da Tao zhi jian

(pronounced *duh dah dow jr jyen*)

Attain the true and ultimate simplicity of The Big Way

This year I was invited to join the International Conference of the Society for Chinese Philosophy at the State University of New York at Buffalo in the United States. I took this opportunity to visit Toronto to meet Zhi Gang and then Vancouver to meet Mrs. Chen. I could see that Zhi Gang has become an extraordinary and world-renowned grandmaster with thousands of students and followers. I learned that he has dedicated himself to travel worldwide spreading healing and teaching in many countries, including India, Japan, the United States, Canada, Taiwan, Australia, Malaysia, and many countries in Europe. In some places, thousands of participants attend his events and workshops. I am so proud of him and so happy for him.

Now I am able to witness the process of Zhi Gang flowing his new book, *Soul Healing Miracles*, which will be published soon. Knowing how many people's lives will be saved and transformed by his new book, I am extremely happy as his teacher. In a moment of great joy, I wrote a special calligraphy to show my appreciation of his extraordinary achievements over the twenty years since I first met him:

靈光救世

Ling Guang Jiu Shi

(pronounced *ling gwahng jeo shr*)

Soul Light Saves the World and Humanity

and

靈光乍閃

Ling Guang Zha Shan

(pronounced *ling gwahng jah shahn*)

Soul Light Explodes and Vibrates

The famous ancient Chinese Confucian philosopher, Xunzi, said 不积跬步, 無以致千里, "Bu Ji Kui Bu, Wu Yi Zhi Qian Li" (pronounced *boo jee kway boo, woo yee jr chyen lee*). This means *every great achievement starts from one small step; with time and constant effort, traverse a thousand miles*. This teaches us that when we make commitments and apply consistent and diligent effort, we can achieve huge goals and fulfill our dreams marvelously.

This is one of the secret keys to Dr. and Master Sha's extraordinary achievements. He started his soul journey unusually early. At age six, he started learning tai chi with a grandmaster. Then he began learning qi gong at age ten. By age twelve, he became a serious practitioner of Shaolin martial arts, including boxing and sticks. In his twenties, he began studying traditional Chinese medicine and unique acupuncture techniques with several grandmaster teachers in these fields and developed his own special acupuncture technique that produced great healing results. In his thirties, he became my devoted disciple to study *I Ching* with me. Before his mid-life, he had already immersed himself in and become a master of all these wonderful ancient Asian arts. In his forties, he began to integrate ancient sacred culture and wisdom of Xiu Lian (pronounced *sheo lyen*), which is the totality of the spiritual journey, with the essences of traditional Chinese medicine and modern allopathic medicine.

He purified his soul, heart, mind, and body very deeply with extreme dedication, perseverance, and commitment. As a result, he created Soul

Mind Body Medicine, which is one of the greatest achievements in his life to date. It has benefited hundreds of thousands of people worldwide.

Dr. and Master Sha has devoted his whole life to learn and improve so that he can be a better servant of the Divine in order to serve humanity and Mother Earth. He has vigorously and courageously forged ahead, seeking new sacred wisdom from Heaven and tirelessly working to share it with all of humanity. Not only am I extremely proud of all his extraordinary achievements over the years, but I am also deeply touched and moved by his indescribable big love, big compassion, and the bright light within his heart to help and serve all lives. Therefore, I am very happy to write this introduction to his *Soul Healing Miracles* book.

Sincerely,

劉大鈞
Professor Liu Da Jun
Shandong University
Chief Editor, Studies of ZhouYi
President, Chinese ZhouYi Society
Board Member, Chinese Ancient Philosophy Research Center
Member, Central Research Institute of Culture and History
Jinan, Shandong province, China
August 2013

You have just read an English translation of Prof. Liu Da Jun's introduction to this book.

The following eight pages are the introduction as originally written by Prof. Liu in Chinese.

序

二十年前中国七省文化代表团来加

拿大举办中国文化展览。沙志刚渡

有国务院报道中涉知我作为山东省

文化顾问来到加拿大的消息。于是专

程前来宾馆见我。交谈中我发现其为人

旷情真挚，率性至真，且思路敏捷，谈

言练达，我们聊的极为欣悦。在此情况下，

志刚提出要拜我为师，跟我学习易经。

我見其中醫、針灸皆師從名家、學

有專長、於是我高興地收其為弟子、利

用在加拿大的短暫逗留、我向他傳授了易、

道之知柔知剛、知微知彰、知圓知方、知

行知藏的變化之要、教學中我發現志

剛才思縱橫、天資甚惡高、對易之何以

及易道之源、何以載索靜精微為易之精

要、皆能淳出自己獨見、我甬之欣然

從此我們保持著聯系、之後數年我又
到加拿大時、志剛的中醫、特別是針灸史已
在加國名聲、甚高、此是我遇沙氏神針
福澤億民、以贊之、這時事業上已顯
俱規模的沙志剛又介紹蔡銀子小姐拜
我為師、由於志剛的減、他已於靈
脫身醫學登堂入室、先儒云減者
天之道、思減专人之道、古人已將減

納入天道范疇、因為誠足有能量的、

"精誠所至，金石為開"、誠能動天地、至誠

之道可以前知。二零零年志剛利用回家

過春節之機喜程興蔡銀子小姐到濟南

看望我、蔡小姐向我介紹了志剛愛看病的種

夕神速、志剛又将他唱的心靈之歌碟帶給我、

他那富有磁性的嘹亮渾厚歌聲給我

傳來特殊氣塲興境界、使我如同回到孩

提時代、常々隨歌起舞，并與志剛同唱，因而

身心得到極大愉悅、故我撰聯以贊之：

闡玄天妙語

浮大道至簡

今年我又利用到美國布法羅大學參加國際

中國哲學會年會之機到加拿大多倫多興邁

歇華更望他們二人、在多倫多期間我見

到志剛已有弟子千餘人從學、并到印度，日

本、美国、欧洲诸国及台湾地区讲
学、聽講者常至數千乃至數萬人
已卓然成一代大家、今又睹其弘著"靈
治療奇迹系列"即将付梓問世,普救
眾生,遂欣然命筆为其新著題
靈光救世""靈光乍见"以彰艾精.
先儒云"不積跬步,无以致千里"、
动志剛毅,能有今日成就,是因艾六岁

学练太极功法，十岁从成人修练气功，十二岁以学习少林拳及其棍法、二十岁学中医，后又从名家研攻针灸。年过而立又没我读书，因自小受中国传统文化的润泽，因而步入四十岁之后，即把中国古老的神秘文化及其修练智慧与中西医西学精萃相结合，经反複苦修，终成正果开创灵脈身医以学而

獲今日盛譽、二十餘年秉志剛奮

勇精進、求知不懈的精神及大愛

大慈悲的光明心靈令我非常

感動,遂於遲辭之後再制短文

此上以為此書之序。

劉大鈞 二〇一三年七月廿八日

書於加拿大多倫多賓館

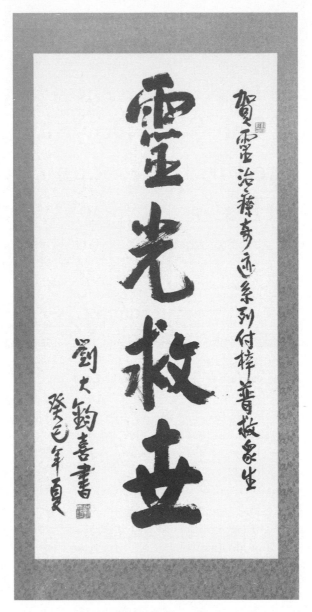

Figure 1. Ling Guang Jiu Shi Calligraphy by Prof. Liu Da Jun
Soul Light Saves the World
*Congratulations on publishing the Soul Healing Miracles Series
to serve all people.*

How to Receive the Divine and Tao Soul Downloads Offered in the Books of the Soul Healing Miracles Series

THE BOOKS of the Soul Healing Miracles Series are unique. The Divine and Tao are downloading their soul treasures to readers as they read these books. Every book in the Soul Healing Miracles Series will include Divine or Tao Soul Downloads that have been pre-programmed. When you read the appropriate paragraphs and pause for a minute, divine or Tao permanent soul mind body treasures will be transmitted to your soul.

In April 2005 the Divine told me to "leave Divine Soul Downloads to history." I thought, "A human being's life is limited. Even if I live a long, long life, I will go back to Heaven one day. How can I leave Divine Soul Downloads to history?"

In the beginning of 2008, as I was editing the paperback edition of *Soul Wisdom*, the first book in my Soul Power Series, the Divine suddenly told me, "Zhi Gang, offer my downloads within this book. I will preprogram my downloads in the book. Any reader can receive them as he or she reads the special pages." At the moment the Divine gave me this direction, I understood how I could leave Divine Soul Downloads to history.

The Divine is the creator and spiritual father and mother of all souls.

Tao is the Source and creator of countless planets, stars, galaxies, and universes. Tao is The Way of all life. Tao is the universal principles and laws.

At the end of 2008 Tao chose me as a servant, vehicle, and channel to offer Tao Soul Downloads. I was extremely honored. I have offered countless Divine and Tao Soul Downloads to humanity and wan ling (all souls) in countless planets, stars, galaxies, and universes.

Preprogrammed Divine and Tao Soul Downloads are permanently stored within this book. Preprogrammed Divine or Tao Soul Downloads are permanently stored within every book in the Soul Healing Miracles Series. If people read this book thousands of years from now, they will still receive the Divine Soul Downloads. As long as this book exists and is read, readers will receive the Divine Soul Downloads.

Allow me to explain further. The Divine has placed a permanent blessing within certain paragraphs in this book. These blessings allow you to receive Divine Soul Downloads as permanent gifts to your soul. Because these divine treasures reside with your soul, you can access them twenty-four hours a day—as often as you like, wherever you are—for healing, blessing, and life transformation.

It is very easy to receive the Divine and Tao Soul Downloads in the books of the Soul Healing Miracles Series. After you read the special paragraphs where they are preprogrammed, close your eyes. Receive the special download. It is also easy to apply these divine and Tao treasures. After you receive a Divine or Tao Soul Download, I will immediately show you how to apply it for healing, blessing, and life transformation.

You have free will. If you are not ready to receive a Divine or Tao Soul Download, simply tell the Divine and Tao *I am not ready to receive this gift*. You can then continue to read the special download paragraphs, but you will not receive the gifts they contain. The Divine and Tao do not offer Divine and Tao Soul Downloads to those who are not ready or not willing to receive their treasures. However, the moment you are ready, you can simply go back to the relevant paragraphs and tell the Divine and Tao *I am ready*. You will then receive the stored special downloads when you reread the paragraphs.

The Divine and Tao have agreed to offer specific Divine and Tao Soul Downloads in these books to all readers who are willing to receive them. The Divine and Tao have unlimited treasures. However, you can receive only the ones designated in these pages. Please do not ask for different or additional gifts. It will not work.

After receiving and practicing with the Divine and Tao Soul Downloads in these books, you could experience remarkable healing results in your spiritual, mental, emotional, and physical bodies. You could receive incredible blessings for your relationships. You could receive financial blessings and all kinds of other blessings.

Divine and Tao Soul Downloads are unlimited. There can be a Divine or Tao Soul Download for anything that exists in the physical world. The reason for this is very simple. *Everything has a soul, mind, and body.* A house has a soul, mind, and body. The Divine and Tao can download a soul to your house that can transform its energy. The Divine and Tao can download a soul to your business that can transform your business. If you are wearing a ring, that ring has a soul. If the Divine downloads a new divine soul to your ring, you can ask the divine soul in your ring to offer divine healing and blessing.

I am honored to have been chosen as a servant of humanity, the Divine, and Tao to offer Divine and Tao Soul Downloads. For the rest of my life, I will continue to offer Divine and Tao Soul Downloads. I will offer more and more of them. I will offer Divine and Tao Soul Downloads for every aspect of every life.

I am honored to be a servant of Divine and Tao Soul Downloads.

What to Expect After You Receive Divine and Tao Soul Downloads

Divine and Tao Soul Downloads are new souls created from the heart of the Divine or the heart of Tao. When these souls are transmitted, you may feel a strong vibration. For example, you could feel warm or excited. Your body could shake a little. You may not feel anything. Advanced spiritual beings with an open Third Eye can actually see a huge golden, rainbow, purple, or crystal light soul enter your body.

These divine and Tao souls are your yin companions[1] for life. They will stay with your soul forever. Even after your physical life ends, these divine and Tao treasures will continue to accompany your soul into your next life and all of your future lives. In these books, I will teach you how to invoke these divine and Tao souls anytime, anywhere to give

---

[1] A yang companion is a physical being, such as a family member, friend, or pet. A yin companion is a soul companion without a physical form, such as your spiritual fathers and mothers in Heaven.

you divine and Tao healing or blessing in this life. You also can invoke these souls to radiate out to offer divine and Tao healing or blessing to others. These divine and Tao souls have extraordinary abilities to heal, bless, and transform. If you develop advanced spiritual abilities in your next life, you will discover that you have these divine or Tao souls with you. You will then be able to invoke these souls in the same way in your future lifetimes to heal, bless, and transform every aspect of your life.

It is a great honor to have a divine or Tao soul downloaded to your own soul. The divine or Tao soul is a pure soul without bad karma. The divine or Tao soul carries divine and Tao healing and blessing abilities. The download does not have any side effects. You are given love and light with divine and Tao frequency. You are given divine and Tao abilities to serve yourself and others. Therefore, humanity is extremely honored that the Divine and Tao are offering Divine and Tao Soul Downloads. I am extremely honored to be a servant of the Divine, of Tao, of you, of all humanity, and of all souls to offer Divine and Tao Soul Downloads. I cannot thank the Divine and Tao enough. I cannot thank you, all humanity, and all souls enough for the opportunity to serve.

Thank you. Thank you. Thank you.

How to Receive Maximum Benefits from My Books

LIKE MANY PEOPLE WORLDWIDE, you may have read my books before. You may be reading my books for the first time. When you start to read my books, you may realize quickly that they include many practices for healing the spiritual, mental, emotional, and physical bodies, as well as for transforming relationships and finances. I teach the Four Power Techniques to transform all life. I will summarize each of my Four Power Techniques in one sentence:

BODY POWER: Where you put your hands is where you receive benefits for healing and rejuvenation.

SOUL POWER: Apply Say Hello Healing and Blessing to invoke the inner souls of your body, systems, organs, cells, DNA, and RNA; and invoke the outer souls of the Divine, Tao, Heaven, Mother Earth, and countless planets, stars, galaxies, and universes, as well as all kinds of spiritual fathers and mothers on Mother Earth and in all layers of Heaven, to request their help for your healing, rejuvenation, and transformation of relationships and finances.

MIND POWER: Where you put your mind, using creative visualization, is where you receive benefits for healing, rejuvenation, and transformation of relationships and finances.

SOUND POWER: What you chant is what you become.

My books are unique. Each one includes many practices with chanting (Sound Power). I repeat some chants again and again in the books of my Soul Power Series and in this book. It is most important for you, dear reader, to avoid thinking *I already know this*, and then quickly read through the text without doing the practices. That would be a big mistake. You will miss some of the most important parts of my teaching: the practices.

Imagine you are in a workshop. When the teacher leads you to meditate or chant, you do it. Otherwise, you will not receive the benefits from the meditation and chanting. People are familiar with the ancient Chinese martial art and teaching of kung fu. A kung fu master spends an entire lifetime to develop power. In one sentence:

Time is kung fu and kung fu is time.

You have to spend time to chant and meditate. Remember the one-sentence secret for Sound Power: *What you chant is what you become*. Therefore, when you read the practices where I am leading you to chant, please do them. Do not pass them by. The practices are jewels of my teaching. Practice is necessary to transform and bring success to any aspect of your life, including health, relationships, finances, intelligence, and more.

There is a renowned spiritual practice in Buddhism. Millions of people throughout history have chanted *Na Mo A Mi Tuo Fo* (pronounced *nah maw ah mee twaw faw*). A Mi Tuo Fo is a buddha's name (Amitabha in Sanskrit). Many practitioners chant only this one mantra. They could chant *Na Mo A Mi Tuo Fo* for hours a day for their entire life. It is a great practice. If you are upset, chant *Na Mo A Mi Tuo Fo*. If you are sick, chant *Na Mo A Mi Tuo Fo*. If you are weak, chant *Na Mo A Mi Tuo Fo*. If you are emotional, chant *Na Mo A Mi Tuo Fo*. If you have relationship challenges, chant *Na Mo A Mi Tuo Fo*. If you have financial challenges, chant *Na Mo A Mi Tuo Fo*. Chanting is transforming but to transform life takes time. You must understand this spiritual wisdom so that you will practice chanting and meditation more and more. The more you practice, the more healing and life transformation you could receive.

For success in any profession, one must study and practice again and again to gain mastery. My teaching is soul healing and soul transformation of every aspect of life. You must apply the Four Power Techniques again and again to receive maximum benefits from soul healing and soul transformation for every aspect of your life.

If you go into the condition of *what you chant is what you become*, a wonderful healing result may come suddenly, and transformation of relationships and finances may follow. "Aha!" moments may come. "Wow!" moments may come.

I bring my workshops and retreats to you in every book. Apply the wisdom. Take time to practice seriously. Chant and meditate using the Four Power Techniques.

My books have another unique aspect: the Divine and Tao offer Soul Mind Body Transplants as you read. Divine and Tao Soul Mind Body Transplants are permanent healing and blessing treasures from the Divine and Tao.

These treasures carry Divine and Tao frequency and vibration, which can transform the frequency and vibration of your health, relationships, finances, intelligence, and more.

These treasures carry Divine and Tao love, which melts all blockages and transforms all life.

These treasures carry Divine and Tao forgiveness, which brings inner joy and inner peace to all life.

These treasures carry Divine and Tao compassion, which boosts energy, stamina, vitality, and immunity of all life.

These treasures carry Divine and Tao light, which heals, prevents sickness, purifies and rejuvenates soul, heart, mind, and body, transforms relationships and finances, increases intelligence, and brings success in every aspect of life.

I summarize and emphasize the two absolutely unique aspects of my books. First, I bring my workshops and retreats to you in my books. Please practice seriously, just as though you were in a workshop with me. Second, as you read, you can receive permanent treasures (Soul Mind Body Transplants) from the Divine and Tao to transform your health, relationships, finances, and more.

Pay great attention to these two unique aspects in order to receive maximum benefits from this book and any of my books.

I wish you will receive maximum benefits from this book to transform every aspect of your life.

Practice. Practice. Practice.

Transform. Transform. Transform.

Enlighten. Enlighten. Enlighten.

Success. Success. Success.

List of Tao (Source) Soul Downloads

List of Figures

Ancient and New Sacred Wisdom, Knowledge, and Practical Techniques for Healing

MILLIONS OF PEOPLE on Mother Earth are searching for ancient secrets, wisdom, knowledge, and practical techniques for healing, rejuvenation, and prolonging life, as well as for transformation of relationships, finances, business, and every aspect of life.

The Soul Healing Miracles Series shares ancient and new sacred wisdom, knowledge, and practical techniques to transform all life. This first book in the series emphasizes healing for the spiritual, mental, emotional, and physical bodies.

I have studied conventional medicine as an MD. I honor conventional medicine. I have studied traditional Chinese medicine as an acupuncturist and herbalist. I honor traditional Chinese medicine. I have studied ancient Chinese energy and spiritual practices, including tai chi, qi gong, kung fu, *I Ching*, and feng shui. I honor each of them. I have studied Zhi Neng Medicine, which is the medicine of the intelligence of the mind and soul. I have studied Body Space Medicine, which is the medicine of the spaces between the organs and between the cells. I honor both of them.

I am extremely blessed to have met and studied with many teachers who are Chinese national treasures. They have taught me ancient and sacred spiritual and energy wisdom, knowledge, and practical techniques.

At age six I met my Wu Dang Chinese master who taught me tai chi. At age ten I met my qi gong master. At age twelve I met my Shaolin Kung Fu master. Later I met the world's top *I Ching* authority, Dr. and Professor Liu Da Jun. I have learned profound sacred wisdom and philosophy of *I Ching* and feng shui from him. I am extremely blessed that he has written a foreword for this book.

In 1993 I met my spiritual father and mentor, Dr. and Master Zhi Chen Guo, the founder of Zhi Neng Medicine and Body Space Medicine. He has taught me profound secrets, wisdom, knowledge, and practical techniques about soul. His teaching has greatly benefited me. He has prepared me to be a divine servant, vehicle, and channel. I am extremely grateful for his teaching.

I also deeply appreciate the teaching from my Peng Zu lineage master, Dr. and Professor Liu De Hua. Peng Zu, who lived to the age of eight hundred eighty, is renowned in China as the "Long Life Star." Peng Zu is the teacher of Lao Zi, author of the revered classic, *Dao De Jing*. Peng Zu's and Prof. Liu's sacred ancient wisdom and practice have deeply benefited my spiritual journey.

A few of my masters wish to remain anonymous. Their profound sacred wisdom and practices have benefited my soul journey beyond words. I cannot honor them enough.

In ancient Chinese spiritual teaching there is a sacred phrase:

Yin shui si yuan

"Yin" literally means *drink*. "Shui" means *water*. "Si" means *to think*. "Yuan" means *source* or *origin*. "Yin shui si yuan" (pronounced *yeen shway sz ywen*) means *when you drink water, think of the source*.

This sacred phrase made me realize deeply in my heart and soul that I could not have grown to where I am today in my spiritual journey and would not have the ancient sacred wisdom, knowledge, techniques, and healing power to transform the lives of others without the teaching of these national treasures. I am honored to share what I have learned. I am your servant.

San Mi (*Three Secrets*)

In this turn of Mother Earth there are historical records dating back thousands of years. We understand that Mother Earth has been in many turns before. Mother Earth has reincarnated many times. Reincarnation is a universal law. I shared in the introduction that the oldest minerals analyzed to date were found in Western Australia and are at least 4.4 billion years old. In the future, scientists could discover much older minerals on Mother Earth.

Time also reincarnates. A new era for Mother Earth and all universes begins every fifteen thousand years. On August 8, 2003 the previous era ended. It was Xia Gu (pronounced *shyah goo*), the *near ancient* era. Archeologists estimate that modern humans have been on Mother Earth for about two hundred thousand years. I received a spiritual message from Heaven that human beings have existed on Mother Earth for much longer than two hundred thousand years. It will take time for scientists to find evidence of this.

Some archaeologists say that symbols found in China carved into 8,600-year-old tortoise shells may be the earliest written words. We do not have enough records from twenty thousand to thirty thousand years ago or even earlier to explain what had happened with humanity on Mother Earth.

From ancient times up to now, one of the biggest treasures that has been left to humanity and given us great benefits is sacred spiritual wisdom and practice. This sacred spiritual wisdom and practice is continually guiding humanity to transform every aspect of their lives. Sacred spiritual wisdom and practice from ancient times up to now can be summarized as *San Mi*. "San Mi" means *three secrets*. I will explain San Mi further.

San Mi includes *Shen Mi*, *Kou Mi*, and *Yi Mi*.

1. Shen Mi—Body Secret

"Shen" means *body*. "Mi" means *secret*. "Shen Mi" (pronounced *shun mee*) means *Body Secret*. If you observe statues and paintings in all kinds of spiritual temples and churches around the world and in every spiritual tradition, the masters, buddhas, and saints apply special hand positions or mudras as well as body positions when they meditate or do spiritual practice. That is Shen Mi, *Body Secret*. There are so many body secrets. Every hand and body position benefits different parts of the body.

Shen Mi can be summarized in one sentence:

Where you put your hands is where you receive the benefits for healing, rejuvenation, and development.

2. Kou Mi—Mouth Secret

"Kou" means *mouth*. "Mi" means *secret*. "Kou Mi" (pronounced *koe mee*) means *Mouth Secret*, which is *chanting mantras*. Mantras are sacred sounds and messages chanted repeatedly for healing and preventing sickness, rejuvenation, prolonging life, and transforming relationships, finances, and every aspect of life.

I will give one example. Billions of people on Mother Earth have learned and continue to learn from Buddhism. One of the most renowned mantras in Buddhist teaching is:

Na Mo A Mi Tuo Fo

"Na Mo" (pronounced *nah maw*) means *revere*. "A Mi Tuo Fo" (pronounced *ah mee twaw faw*) is a buddha's name (Amitabha in Sanskrit). The founder of Buddhism, Shi Jia Mo Ni Fo (pronounced *shr jyah maw nee faw*), also known as Shakyamuni Buddha and Siddhartha Gautama, in the stillness of his meditation found A Mi Tuo Fo, who is an ancient buddha from a long, long time ago. A Mi Tuo Fo was an emperor in ancient times. He abdicated his throne to follow his spiritual master, with the goal of reaching soul enlightenment. A Mi Tuo Fo made forty-eight vows to create *Ji Le Shi Jie*, a spiritual realm in Heaven. "Ji" means *most*. "Le" means *happiness*. "Shi Jie" means *the world*. "Ji Le Shi Jie" (pronounced *jee luh shr jyeh*) means *the world of most happiness*. It is also named the *Pure Land*. This Land has no ego, no anger, no fighting, no jealousy, and no competition. Those who inhabit the Pure Land share love, care, and compassion with each other. They are uplifting their soul journeys higher and higher.

A Mi Tuo Fo's eighteenth vow is the most important of his forty-eight vows. He vowed that if anyone who believes in him and desires to go to his Pure Land chants his name ten times shortly before transitioning from physical life, A Mi Tuo Fo's soul will personally bring this one's soul to his Pure Land. A Mi Tuo Fo has gathered countless buddhas, bodhisattvas, and other high-level souls in his realm to do spiritual practice to advance their soul journeys.

There are three leaders in the Pure Land. They are Guan Yin, the Compassion Buddha, Da Shi Zhi (pronounced *dah shr jr*), the Intelligence Buddha, and A Mi Tuo Fo. Billions of people in history have honored the three of them. The most important spiritual achievement for Buddhists is to go to the Pure Land after physical life ends in order to continue their spiritual journey.

Billions of Buddhists in history have chanted *Na Mo A Mi Tuo Fo*. Why do they chant *Na Mo A Mi Tuo Fo*? The teaching is *to chant Na Mo A Mi Tuo Fo is to become a buddha*.

A human being has two lives: physical life and soul life. Physical life is limited. The soul journey is eternal. The purpose of physical life is to serve the soul journey. Why have billions of people chanted *Na Mo A Mi Tuo Fo*? It is because they love and believe in A Mi Tuo Fo. They want to go to his realm to reach advanced soul enlightenment.

Shi Jia Mo Ni Fo introduced A Mi Tuo Fo to Buddhist followers. Shi Jia Mo Ni Fo taught eighty-four thousand methods to reach enlightenment. One of the most important methods is to *chant a buddha's name to become a buddha*.

When you chant a buddha's name, the buddha's heart is your heart; the buddha's soul is your soul; the buddha's will is your will; and the buddha's mission is your mission. The buddha's heart, soul, will, and mission is the same heart, soul, will, and mission of those who chant the buddha's name with great devotion and dedication. This teaching has benefited billions of people in history. Words are not enough to express the benefit and significance of this teaching and practice.

This teaching can be summarized in one sentence:

**To chant a buddha and become a buddha
is to join with a buddha as One.**

I emphasize that I am not teaching religion. I honor all religions. I honor all kinds of spiritual belief systems. I share this practice to let every reader understand the sacred wisdom and teaching of spiritual practice. Chanting *Na Mo A Mi Tuo Fo* has brought many soul healing miracles for healing and for transformation of relationships, finances, and every aspect of life. Billions of people in history have chanted *Na Mo Guan Shi Yin Pusa*[2] (pronounced *nah maw gwahn shr yeen poo sah*) and *Na Mo Da Shi Zhi Pusa* (pronounced *nah maw dah shr jr poo sah*), to honor the other two leaders of the Pure Land. Chanting these two mantras has also brought many heart-touching and moving stories.

In this book I will release ancient sacred mantras and new sacred mantras that the Divine and The Source have asked me to share with every reader and humanity. When you understand the wisdom, you will chant much more seriously. The benefits are beyond words, thoughts, and comprehension.

Kou Mi can be summarized in one sentence:

What you chant is what you become.

You could find this scientific article, "Scientists Prove DNA Can Be Reprogrammed by Words and Frequencies,"[3] very interesting to understand more about how Kou Mi, which I call Sound Power, works.

You will learn and experience a lot about chanting mantras in this book and in other books of the Soul Healing Miracles Series.

---

[2] "Pusa" (pronounced *poo sah*) means bodhisattva. A bodhisattva is an enlightened being. A buddha is a being who has attained an even higher level of enlightenment.

[3] Grazyna Fosar and Franz Bludorf: http://wakeup-world.com/2011/07/12/scientist-prove-dna-can-be-reprogrammed-by-words-frequencies/

3. Yi Mi—Thinking Secret

"Yi" means *thinking*. "Mi" means *secret*. "Yi Mi" (pronounced *yee mee*) means *thinking secret*. In history billions of people have meditated. To meditate is to train the mind. There are countless ways to meditate in all kinds of spiritual practices. What is the key to meditation?

Some people meditate by visualizing the sun and the moon. Some people meditate by visualizing the Big Dipper. Some people meditate by visualizing a mountain or ocean. Some people meditate by visualizing the Buddha or a holy saint or other spiritual fathers and mothers. Meditation can be summarized in one sentence:

**Meditation is creative visualization: what you visualize
is what you receive blessings from.**

Let me explain this one-sentence secret further. For example, if you visualize Jesus, you connect with Jesus' soul. Jesus' healing power could benefit your healing journey very much. If you visualize Mother Mary, Mother Mary's love could benefit you a lot. If you visualize Guan Yin, Guan Yin's compassion could open your heart further. If you visualize the sun and the moon, you receive the jing qi shen of the sun and the moon. You receive the blessing from whomever or whatever you visualize.

In ancient teaching, to apply one secret is powerful. Shen Mi, Kou Mi, and Yi Mi are each powerful if applied individually. To apply all three secrets together is *extremely* powerful.

Now I will share one sacred practice to apply San Mi, the *three secrets*, together. This is the Compassion Buddha Practice.

I will lead and guide you through two variations. The first is a practice to boost energy, stamina, vitality, immunity, and healing. The second is a practice to open the Third Eye and other spiritual channels.

Boost Energy, Stamina, Vitality, Immunity, and Healing with the Sacred Mantra *Weng Ma Ni Ba Ma Hong*

Shen Mi. *Body Secret.*

Sit up straight on a chair with your back free and clear. Place your hands in the Pyramid Style Hands Position.[4] See figure 2.

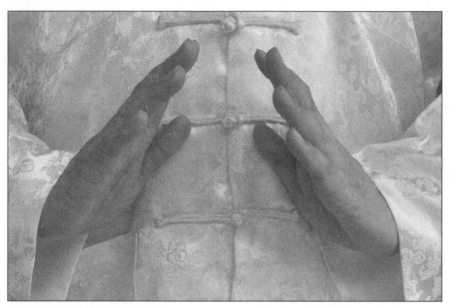

FIGURE 2. Pyramid Style Hands Shen Mi

Kou Mi. *Mouth Secret.*

Chant *Weng Ma Ni Ba Ma Hong*, Guan Yin's six-word enlightenment mantra. This ancient mantra has been chanted by millions of spiritual practitioners throughout history.

> *Weng Ma Ni Ba Ma Hong* (pronounced *wung mah nee bah mah hawng*)

---

[4] Hold both hands in front of you with palms facing each other. Spread the heels of your hands (inner wrists) five to seven inches apart while keeping your fingertips only two or three inches apart. Place both hands around the level of the navel. This is the Pyramid Style Hands Position or Pyramid Style Hands Shen Mi.

Weng Ma Ni Ba Ma Hong
Weng Ma Ni Ba Ma Hong
Weng Ma Ni Ba Ma Hong
Weng Ma Ni Ba Ma Hong
Weng Ma Ni Ba Ma Hong
Weng Ma Ni Ba Ma Hong...

Chant for a minimum of ten minutes. The longer you chant and the more often you chant, the better the results you could receive.

Through soul communication, Guan Yin released the secret to me in 2012 that each word of this sacred mantra resonates and vibrates a specific area inside the body. See figure 3.

Yi Mi. *Thinking Secret.*
Visualize golden light from Heaven pouring into your crown chakra at the top of your head, and down through the seven chakras in the center of your body to your Kun Gong area. Kun Gong (pronounced *kwun gawng*) is a sacred space located behind the navel area that produces Yuan Jing (pronounced *ywen jing*) and Yuan Qi (pronounced *ywen chee*), original jing (matter) and original qi (energy).

I have shared these profound secrets in my books *Tao I: The Way of All Life* and *Tao II: The Way of Healing, Rejuvenation, Longevity, and Immortality*. I will emphasize the essence here.

When a father's sperm and a mother's egg unite, Tao (The Source) gives Yuan Shen to the embryo. "Yuan" means *origin*. "Shen" means *soul*. "Yuan Shen" (pronounced *ywen shun*) means *original soul*. Yuan Shen produces Yuan Qi and Yuan Jing. Yuan Qi is the original energy. Yuan Jing is the original matter. Together, Yuan Qi, Yuan Jing, and Yuan Shen are like the oil in a full oil lamp. They are the true life force for a human being.

Sickness and the aging process gradually deplete Yuan Shen, Yuan Qi, and Yuan Jing. When Yuan Shen, Yuan Qi, and Yuan Jing are exhausted, the oil in one's oil lamp is exhausted, and one's physical life ends.

Generally speaking, a person's Yuan Shen, Yuan Qi, and Yuan Jing cannot be replenished. However, this year, 2013, The Source gave me the honor, authority, and ability to replenish Yuan Shen, Yuan Qi, and

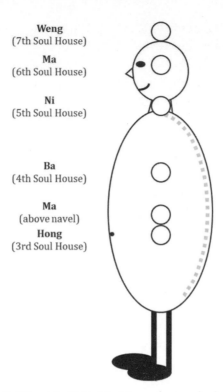

Weng
(7th Soul House)

Ma
(6th Soul House)

Ni
(5th Soul House)

Ba
(4th Soul House)

Ma
(above navel)

Hong
(3rd Soul House)

Figure 3. *Weng Ma Ni Ba Ma Hong* vibrates the body

Yuan Jing. I was in the speechless condition when I received this honor. The significance of this honor is that a bodily system, an organ, or a part of the body can be instantly rejuvenated. The Yuan Shen, Yuan Qi, and Yuan Jing of the system, organ, or part of the body are replenished to a full bottle of oil. Words cannot express the greatest gratitude from my heart and soul to The Source for this honor.

In a few short months I have offered thousands of replenishments of Yuan Shen, Yuan Qi, and Yuan Jing for people around the world. For fifteen weeks this year I traveled to many cities in Canada, the United States, Germany, England, and other countries in Europe to offer this service. Thousands of soul healing miracles have been created by this service. To understand more about my teaching and about soul healing and soul healing results, you can view a video of soul healing miracles at www.drsha.com/soulhealingmiraclesmovie2013.

I explain this to let every reader know the importance of Kun Gong. Kun Gong is a spiritual temple inside the body. It is the sacred place to produce Yuan Qi and Yuan Jing. Generally speaking, Yuan Qi and Yuan Jing cannot be produced by food or physical exercise. Only sacred spiritual practice can replenish Yuan Qi and Yuan Jing little by little.

Chanting *Weng Ma Ni Ba Ma Hong* brings the essence of the energy from Heaven and Mother Earth. It starts at the crown chakra and goes through the chakras to the Kun Gong to fulfill Yuan Qi and Yuan Jing little by little. Therefore, *Weng Ma Ni Ba Ma Hong* is a sacred practice that Guan Yin has left to humanity to empower us to receive blessings for healing, rejuvenation, and prolonging life. I honor Guan Yin's service deeply.

Let us chant for ten minutes more.

> *Weng Ma Ni Ba Ma Hong* (pronounced *wung mah nee bah mah hawng*)
> *Weng Ma Ni Ba Ma Hong*
> *Weng Ma Ni Ba Ma Hong*
> *Weng Ma Ni Ba Ma Hong*
> *Weng Ma Ni Ba Ma Hong*
> *Weng Ma Ni Ba Ma Hong*
> *Weng Ma Ni Ba Ma Hong…*

I have explained how this sacred practice can fulfill Yuan Qi and Yuan Jing to boost energy, stamina, vitality, and immunity; to rejuvenate; and to prolong life. This sacred practice not only brings these benefits; this practice is also for healing. To fulfill Yuan Qi and Yuan Jing little by little is to increase the true life force. The immune system is boosted. Circulation is promoted. Blockages in the chakras could be removed. The healing results could be heart-touching and profound.

Weng Ma Ni Ba Ma Hong has already created hundreds of thousands of soul healing miracles in history.

Practice more and more. Soul healing miracles could be in front of you.

Open Direct Soul Communication and Third Eye Channels with the Sacred Mantra *Weng Ma Ni Ba Ma Hong*

The Third Eye is the spiritual eye. It is located inside the brain. To locate the Third Eye, draw a line from the midpoint between your eyebrows straight up over your forehead to the top of your head. Draw another line over your head connecting the tops of both ears. At the point where these two perpendicular lines cross, go down about three inches inside your head. This is the location of your Third Eye, a cherry-sized energy center, which corresponds with the location of the pineal gland.

To open the Third Eye is to see spiritual images. Why does a person need to open the Third Eye? To open the Third Eye is to understand Heaven, the Divine, and The Source better. To open the Third Eye is to see spiritual images that enable one to gain spiritual wisdom. To open the Third Eye is to understand one's soul journey better. To open the Third Eye is to gain special abilities to guide others to transform their lives.

To open the Third Eye is to open the Third Eye Channel.

Another one of the most important spiritual abilities is the ability to have a conversation with the Divine, Heaven, and The Source. This is called *direct soul communication*. To do this, one must open his or her Direct Soul Communication Channel.

Weng Ma Ni Ba Ma Hong can help open a person's Third Eye and Direct Soul Communication Channel.

I will emphasize some very important guidance again. When you start to read my books, you may realize quickly that they include many practices for healing, rejuvenation, and longevity, as well as for transforming relationships and finances. Do not skip the practices. That would be a big mistake. You will miss some of the most important parts of my teaching: the practices.

Imagine you are in a workshop. When the teacher leads you to meditate or chant, you have to do it. Otherwise, you will not receive the benefits from the meditation and chanting. Every time I lead you in a practice, be sure to do it.

I will now guide you in a practice to open or further open your Third Eye Channel and Direct Soul Communication Channel.

Shen Mi. *Body Secret.*
Sit up straight with your back free and clear. Put your hands in the Open Lotus Hands Position. Place your hands in front of your chest. Gently touch the heels of your hands, your thumbs, and your little fingers together. Open your hands and fingers as though you were holding a beautiful lotus flower with petals and fingers opening upward to Heaven. See figure 4. Slightly close your eyes while looking at the tips of your fingers.

Yi Mi. *Thinking Secret.*
Visualize rainbow light radiating through your heart chakra in the center of your chest and through your Third Eye area in your brain, opening your Direct Soul Communication Channel and Third Eye Channel.

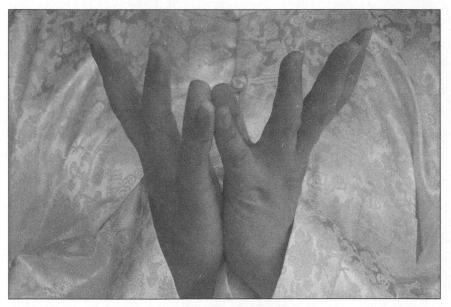

FIGURE 4. Open Lotus Hands Shen Mi

Kou Mi. *Mouth Secret.*
  Chant:

> *Weng Ma Ni Ba Ma Hong*
> *Weng Ma Ni Ba Ma Hong*
> *Weng Ma Ni Ba Ma Hong*
> *Weng Ma Ni Ba Ma Hong*
> *Weng Ma Ni Ba Ma Hong*
> *Weng Ma Ni Ba Ma Hong*
> *Weng Ma Ni Ba Ma Hong…*

Chant for at least ten minutes. The longer and the more often you chant, the faster and wider you could open your Direct Soul Communication and Third Eye Channels.

We have practiced chanting the sacred mantra *Weng Ma Ni Ba Ma Hong* to boost energy, stamina, vitality, immunity, and healing, as well as to open the Direct Soul Communication Channel and Third Eye Channel. After learning the techniques you need to practice a lot on your own. This sacred practice has benefited millions of people in history. I wish for you to receive much more benefit by more practice.

Jing Qi Shen (*Matter, Energy, Soul*)

In ancient spiritual teaching there is profound wisdom that everyone and everything in the universe consists of jing qi shen. "Jing" means *matter*. "Qi" (pronounced *chee*) means *energy*. "Shen" (pronounced *shun*) means *soul*. There are thousands of spiritual and energy practices to develop jing qi shen.

The body is made of jing qi shen. A system is made of jing qi shen. An organ is made of jing qi shen. A cell is made of jing qi shen. DNA and RNA are made of jing qi shen.

Conventional medicine focuses on matter. Blood tests measure biochemical changes inside the cells. CT scans and MRIs detect growths inside the body. Surgery removes matter from the body, including cysts, tumors, stones, and more. Medications adjust the body's matter.

Traditional Chinese medicine focuses on qi. Qi is vital energy and life force. *The Yellow Emperor's Internal Classic*, the ancient authority book of traditional Chinese medicine, states: *If qi flows, one is healthy. If qi is blocked, one is sick.* This theory has guided traditional Chinese medicine for five thousand years. Removing energy blockages for healing has served millions of people throughout history. Traditional Chinese medicine uses herbs, acupuncture, and Chinese massage to promote the flow of qi for healing.

Several years ago, the Divine guided me to create Soul Mind Body Medicine and soul healing. From my more than forty years of energy and spiritual study, together with my study of medicine to become an MD and a doctor of traditional Chinese medicine, I have realized that soul, mind, and body can work together. Conventional medicine and traditional Chinese medicine can work together also.

Conventional medicine focuses on matter inside the cells. Traditional Chinese medicine and many other healing modalities focus on the energy between cells. Soul healing focuses on the soul.

A soul is a golden light being. Soul is spirit. Soul is message. Soul is the essence of life. Soul is the boss of a human being.

The foundational wisdom and practice of soul healing can be summarized in one sentence:

Heal the soul first; then healing of the mind and body will follow.

Now I am releasing another profound one-sentence secret that people have not realized enough or at all:

**When a person gets sick, the soul gets sick first;
then sickness of the mind and body follows.**

For example, before a growth such as a cyst, tumor, or cancer appears in the physical body, the soul of the organ or part of the body is blocked. Soul is *message.* The growth message happens at the invisible level. If this message is not cleared, a physical growth appears.

Because the soul is the boss of the mind and body, sickness starts at the soul level. Then it moves to the mind and body levels. Healing also starts at the soul level. Then the mind and body levels follow. Therefore, the Divine guided me to create Soul Mind Body Medicine. Millions of people speak about body, mind, and spirit. Soul Mind Body Medicine emphasizes that the leader among the soul, mind, and body is the soul.

Every human being has a soul, mind, and body. Soul mind body is jing qi shen. Shen includes soul and mind. Body includes qi (energy) and jing (matter). A bodily system, such as the cardiovascular system or the digestive system, has a soul, mind, and body. Every cell and every DNA and RNA has a soul, mind, and body or jing qi shen. Everyone and everything has a soul, mind, and body or jing qi shen.

Soul healing states that all sickness is due to soul, mind, and body blockages. Soul blockages are due to negative karma. Mind blockages include negative mind-sets, attitudes, and beliefs, as well as ego and attachments. Body blockages are blockages of energy and matter.

To heal is to remove soul, mind, and body blockages. Soul healing removes soul, mind, and body blockages. The techniques are very simple. In fact, they could be too simple to believe. I ask that you keep an open mind and try them. Like thousands of others, you could experience a soul healing miracle.

Soul Mind Body Medicine comes from ancient sacred wisdom of jing qi shen. Einstein's renowned formula, $E=mc^2$, explained the relationship between energy and matter. It does not include the soul.

Soul Mind Body Medicine includes the soul. What I want to share with every reader and humanity is that we have to involve the soul in healing. Thousands of years ago people knew that everything is made of jing qi shen or soul, mind, and body. Soul is the boss of the mind and body. If we do not involve the soul or remove soul blockages, many sicknesses cannot be transformed.

Soul Mind Body Medicine emphasizes soul healing as one of the top healing methods. To remove soul mind body blockages is to heal. I deeply appreciate the ancient wisdom of *jing qi shen*. I deeply appreciate that the Divine and Tao have guided me to create Soul Mind Body Medicine. In 2006 I wrote the book *Soul Mind Body Medicine: A Complete Soul Healing System for Optimum Health and Vitality*. I wish Soul Mind Body Medicine can serve humanity further and further in the future.

I am honored to share soul healing miracle stories throughout this book. May they inspire you to apply the wisdom, knowledge, and practical techniques to create your own soul healing miracles. I wish you great success on your healing, rejuvenation, and transformation journey.

Stage four prostate, lung, and bone cancer healed

In 2010 I was told I had stage 4 cancer of the prostate, lungs, and bones. I had all kinds of tests and every test—biopsy, chest x-ray, bone scan, and pelvic MRI—came back worse than before. My doctor said that I couldn't be helped; I wasn't a candidate for surgery, radiation, or chemotherapy because my cancer was so advanced.

My friend emailed me about an event with Master Sha and said I should go to this event. I did. Master Sha was very gracious and extremely generous to offer me Karma Cleansing, Soul Mind Body Transplants, and other blessings. This was on October 28, 2010. I wasn't exactly sure what was happening, but the next day my urinary symptoms were greatly reduced and they never came back.

Master Sha also gifted me very generously with the 10-day Tao Retreat in Estes Park, Colorado. At the very end of the event, Master Sha gave me more healing. It was very profound. He gave me chanting to do, which I did. This treatment was on November 15. By November 22 my PSA (prostate-specific antigen), which had been 266 (anything above 4 is alarming), went all the way down to 1.

For one year, my PSA stayed low and then it started to come up again. My other tests were going very well: chest x-ray, MRI, and bone scan. Everything was improving. Master Sha offered me healing blessings again and immediately my PSA just dropped like a rock. That treatment was on Monday and the test was only four days later. It went from 18 to 6. Another one month later it was down to 1.8. My lungs are all clear. The tumors were so numerous you couldn't count them. There were hundreds. That was all clear after that Tao retreat. The bones are all clear as well, I think.

The doctor's interpretation of my improvement is that the chemotherapy must be working. I did no chemotherapy!

I am very grateful to Master Sha.

J. C.
Boulder, Colorado, U.S.A.

We tried everything to heal my child's asthma and eczema

My son has suffered with many health issues since he was six months old. He developed severe eczema, his face would redden, and he would develop hives all over his body. He developed allergies to food, the environment, to dust, gluten—everything. You name it. He also had asthma. We made so many trips to the children's hospital. Countless trips. My husband and I spent so many nights at the hospital. They were very, very tough times.

We have been to many practitioners, including naturopaths and traditional Chinese medicine practitioners, and tried ear acupressure, needle acupressure, and more. We tried everything. You name it, we tried it. Everyone said this will heal him. Nothing helped. It cost so much money.

Two years ago we met Master Sha. My son received karma cleansing and other soul healing blessings and his eczema started to improve. I chanted for him. Since almost two years now his eczema is completely gone. With Master Sha's blessing he is healed.

Last year we came to Master Sha's retreat again and he gave my son more blessings. And now his asthma is completely gone too. He doesn't have to carry his inhaler with him anymore. We travel everywhere so that's perfect. The only thing left is some allergies and with Master Sha's blessings that too will be gone one day soon.

I am so thankful to Master Sha and the Divine. We are ever, ever grateful.

J. J.
Canada

This form of healing is revolutionary

I am a psychologist on Vancouver Island on the coast of British Columbia. In May 2010 I came across a book called The Power of Soul *by Dr. and Master Zhi Gang Sha, and it happened to come at a perfect time for me. We were taking a five-day holiday on the west coast, so I could just sit, read, and walk on the beach all day. What I learned in the book spoke to me, even though many of the teachings were not familiar. I just felt the rightness of it.*

I participated in Master Sha's webcast a month later and he offered a healing blessing for an organ or system, so I chose liver. That blessing created profound transformation in my health. I had been seeing medical doctors and health practitioners of all kinds for twenty-five years for help with headaches and fatigue. The Soul Mind Body Transplant for the liver completely transformed my health, my energy, and my life.

This form of healing is revolutionary. I invite you all to try it and experience just how brilliant this is!

Mary Louise Reilly
North Saanich, British Columbia

Five Elements

In traditional Chinese medicine, Five Elements is one of the most important theories and practices. In colleges of traditional Chinese medicine there are very deep teachings on the Five Elements. I teach soul healing. I will not explain the Five Elements in too much detail here. Most important, I will share practical techniques to help you create your own soul healing miracles.

Five Elements is one of the major universal laws. Its significance and power cannot be emphasized enough.

The Five Elements of nature (Wood, Fire, Earth, Metal, Water) summarize and categorize the internal organs, sensory organs, bodily tissues and fluids, emotional body, and more. See figure 5.

Five Elements theory has guided millions of people in history to heal sickness and to rejuvenate soul, heart, mind, and body.

Systems, organs, and cells can all be categorized into the Five Elements. Balancing the Five Elements is one of the keys to healing in traditional Chinese medicine.

Expanding the wisdom, there are countless planets in the universe. They can be categorized into Wood planets, Fire planets, Earth planets, Metal planets, and Water planets.

Countless stars, galaxies, and universes can also be categorized into the Five Elements. Balancing the Five Elements is one of the keys to healing for countless planets, stars, galaxies, and universes.

The Five Elements are Wood, Fire, Earth, Metal, and Water.

Element	Yin Organ	Yang Organ	Body Tissue	Body Fluid	Sense	Unbalanced Emotion	Balanced Emotion
Wood	Liver	Gallbladder	Tendons Nails	Tears	Eyes Sight	Anger	Patience
Fire	Heart	Small Intestine	Blood Vessels	Sweat	Tongue Taste	Depression Anxiety Excitability	Joy
Earth	Spleen	Stomach	Muscles	Saliva	Mouth Lips Speech	Worry	Love Compassion
Metal	Lung	Large Intestine	Skin	Mucus	Nose Smell	Grief Sadness	Courage
Water	Kidney	Urinary Bladder	Bones Joints	Urine	Ears Hearing	Fear	Calmness

FIGURE 5. Five Elements

Wood Element

The Wood element includes the liver, gallbladder, eyes, and tendons in the physical body, anger in the emotional body, and more.

Fire Element

The Fire element includes the heart, small intestine, tongue, and all blood vessels in the physical body, anxiety and depression in the emotional body, and more.

Earth Element

The Earth element includes the spleen, stomach, mouth, lips, gums, teeth, and muscles in the physical body, worry in the emotional body, and more.

Metal Element

The Metal element includes the lungs, large intestine, nose, and skin in the physical body, sadness and grief in the emotional body, and more.

Element	Finger	Taste	Color	Weather	Season	Direction	Phase	Energy
Wood	Index	Sour	Green	Windy	Spring	East	New Yang	Generative
Fire	Middle	Bitter	Red	Hot	Summer	South	Full Yang	Expansive
Earth	Thumb	Sweet	Yellow	Damp	Change of seasons	Central	Yin/Yang Balance	Stabilizing
Metal	Ring	Hot	White	Dry	Autumn	West	New Yin	Contracting
Water	Little	Salty	Blue	Cold	Winter	North	Full Yin	Conserving

FIGURE 5. Five Elements

Water Element

The Water element includes the kidneys, urinary bladder, ears, and bones in the physical body, fear in the emotional body, and more.

The Five Elements have the following relationships:

- generating
- controlling
- over-controlling
- reverse controlling

The *generating* relationship can be understood as the mother-son relationship. The mother gives birth to the son and feeds the son. The mother generates and nourishes the son. There are five mother-son pairs within the Five Elements:

- Wood generates (is the mother of) Fire.
- Fire generates Earth.

- Earth generates Metal.
- Metal generates Water.
- Water generates Wood.

See figure 6. These relationships can be seen in the natural world, where wood ignites to start a fire, a fire produces ash, earth can be mined for metal, metal carries water (as in a bucket or a pipe), and plants grow from spring rain.

Applying this to the organs of the body, a healthy mother organ nourishes the son organ. Therefore, a liver (Wood element) with balanced soul, energy, and matter (shen qi jing) and without blockages will fully nourish the soul, energy, and matter of the heart (Fire element). In the same way, a healthy heart will nourish the spleen (Earth element); a healthy spleen will nourish the lungs (Metal element); healthy lungs

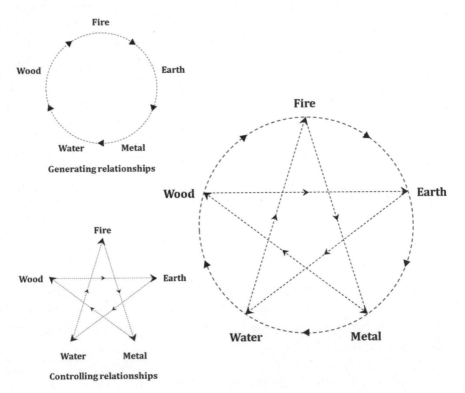

FIGURE 6. Generating and controlling relationships of Five Elements

will nourish the kidneys (Water element); and healthy kidneys will nourish the liver (Wood element).

The generating or mother-son relationships among the Five Elements are extremely important.

The *controlling* relationship shows the order of dominance or control among the Five Elements:

- Wood controls Earth.
- Earth controls Water.
- Water controls Fire.
- Fire controls Metal.
- Metal controls Wood.

See figure 6. In the natural world, wood draws nutrients from earth, earth dams water, water puts out fire, fire melts metal, and metal chops wood.

The *over-controlling* and *reverse controlling* relationships are unbalanced relationships that can be used to describe and explain pathological conditions in the organs of the body. These relationships and conditions are caused by soul mind body or message energy matter blockages.

Five Elements theory can be used to guide us on how to balance the physical body, emotional body, mental body, and spiritual body. It can be applied to balance nature. It can help balance planets, stars, galaxies, and universes.

Major Functions of the Five Elements

Another major theory and core teaching of traditional Chinese medicine is named *zang fu*. "Zang" (pronounced *dzahng*) means *viscera*. "Fu" (pronounced *foo*) means *bowels*. Zang fu includes five zang organs, six fu organs, and "extraordinary" organs.

The five zang organs are the liver, heart, spleen, lungs, and kidneys. Five of the six fu organs are the paired organs of the zang organs. They belong to the Five Elements. They are as follows:

- Wood element—liver (zang), gallbladder (fu)
- Fire element—heart (zang), small intestine (fu)

- Earth element—spleen (zang), stomach (fu)
- Metal element—lungs (zang), large intestine (fu)
- Water element—kidneys (zang), urinary bladder (fu)

San Jiao (pronounced *sahn jee-yow*) is the sixth fu organ. "San" means *three*. "Jiao" means *area*. The San Jiao is the largest fu organ, although it is not an actual organ itself. It is the space inside the body to hold all of the internal organs. San Jiao is divided into Upper Jiao, Middle Jiao, and Lower Jiao. The Upper Jiao is the area above the diaphragm, which includes the heart and lungs. The Middle Jiao is the space in the body between the diaphragm and the level of the navel. It includes the pancreas, stomach, and spleen. The Lower Jiao is the space in the body from the level of the navel down to the genital area; it includes the small and large intestines, urinary bladder, kidneys, reproductive organs, sexual organs, and liver. The liver is physically located in the Middle Jiao but traditional Chinese medicine believes that the liver and kidneys have the same source and a close relationship. Therefore, the liver is included in the Lower Jiao.

The extraordinary organs include the brain, bone marrow, bones, and uterus.

In this book I will introduce only the physiological functions and the pathological changes of the five zang organs: liver, heart, spleen, lungs, and kidneys. They are the authority organs of the Five Elements. As I have shared earlier, the main components of the Five Elements in the body are as follows:

- Wood element—liver (zang), gallbladder (fu), eyes, tendons, and anger in the emotional body
- Fire element—heart (zang), small intestine (fu), tongue, blood vessels, and depression and anxiety in the emotional body
- Earth element—spleen (zang), stomach (fu), muscles, mouth, lips, teeth, gums, and worry in the emotional body
- Metal element—lungs (zang), large intestine (fu), skin, nose, and sadness and grief in the emotional body
- Water element—kidneys (zang), urinary bladder (fu), ears, bones, and fear in the emotional body

The wisdom of five-thousand-year-old traditional Chinese medicine about zang fu is extremely profound. Every reader could understand the body much more.

After sharing this profound wisdom, I will release new soul healing techniques and methods for the Five Elements and zang fu for the first time. I have introduced soul healing for the Five Elements in books of my Soul Power Series. In this book I will go deeper into soul healing for the Five Elements and the internal organs.

Because the liver, heart, spleen, lungs, and kidneys are the authority organs for the Five Elements, I will focus on explaining these five organs and how to do soul healing for them. The six fu organs and the extraordinary organs (brain, bone marrow, bones, and uterus) will receive soul healing benefits automatically because five of them are yin-yang pairs that are closely related. To do soul healing for any one of the five major organs will help heal everything associated with its element. That is the purpose of including this teaching in the book.

It is important to know that the concept of the organs differs between modern allopathic medicine and traditional Chinese medicine. The physiological functions of an organ in traditional Chinese medicine may include the functions of a few organs in modern allopathic medicine. The functions of one organ in modern allopathic medicine may be spread across the functions of several zang fu organs in traditional Chinese medicine. Both medicines are important. They each give us wisdom and offer great benefits, but you should know they are different as you read this book.

The common nature of the five zang organs is to produce, transform, and store essential substances such as essences, qi, blood, and body fluids. The common nature of the six fu organs is to receive, transmit, and digest water and food; and then excrete the waste.

As I explain the major functions of the Five Elements in traditional Chinese medicine, I won't include great detail. If you want to study the Five Elements further, many textbooks of traditional Chinese medicine are available. I am simply providing a basic listing of the key functions of every major organ. Most important, I am sharing soul healing secrets, wisdom, knowledge, and practical techniques to self-heal the

Five Element internal organs, sense organs, body tissues, and emotional body.

I will concentrate on the authority organs of the Five Elements: liver, heart, spleen, lungs, and kidneys. The other organs are important also. It is important to know that when you offer soul healing and rejuvenation to an authority organ of the Five Elements, the rest of the organs belonging to that element will receive benefits simultaneously. The emotional imbalances belonging to that element will also receive benefits simultaneously.

For example, the liver is the authority organ of the Wood element. The Wood element includes the gallbladder, eyes, and tendons in the physical body, and anger in the emotional body. When you do soul healing for your liver, the other organs (gallbladder, eyes), tissues (tendons), and emotional imbalances (anger) in the Wood element will also receive healing and rejuvenation. The same is true for the other four elements.

Now I will explain the key functions of each of the authority organs of the Five Elements.

Liver

The liver is located in the right upper abdomen under the diaphragm. The liver is the zang (authority) organ of the Wood element. The fu organ of the Wood element is the gallbladder. "Zang organ" means *yin organ*. "Fu organ" means *yang organ*. The meridians of the liver and gallbladder are internally and externally related.

1. **Storing and Regulating Blood**
    Normal conditions: When the human body is resting or sleeping, the body needs less blood. Most of the blood remains in the liver. When the physical body is doing physical labor or vigorous movement, the body needs more blood. The liver will release its stored blood to satisfy the needs generated by the activities of the body.
    Abnormal conditions: If the liver's storing and regulating the blood does not function well, the following unhealthy conditions could result: blurred vision, spasms or convulsions of the tendons and muscles, lack of smooth movement of the four extremities, reduction or even stoppage of menstrual blood flow.

2. **Regulating and Maintaining the Flow of Qi and Blood**
   This liver function includes three aspects:

   a) **Regulating emotions**. The heart is the key organ to house the mind and emotions. The liver also affects the emotions.
   Normal conditions: If the liver regulates and maintains free flow of qi and blood well, one feels happy, calm, peaceful, harmonized, and more.
   Abnormal conditions: If the liver does not regulate and maintain the free flow of qi and blood well, the following unhealthy conditions could result: depression, anxiety, weeping, paranoia, belching, headache, dizziness, insomnia, impatience, irritability, agitation, and more.

   b) **Assisting Digestion and Absorption of Food**
   Normal conditions: If the liver regulates and maintains free flow of qi and blood well, it will assist the spleen in sending food essence and water up, support the stomach in sending food contents down, and support the secretion of bile so that the functions of digestion and absorption are normal.
   Abnormal conditions: If the liver does not help digestion and absorption well, the following unhealthy conditions could result: poor appetite, indigestion, diarrhea, bitter taste in mouth, jaundice, constipation, and more.

   c) **Maintaining Free Flow of Qi and Blood**
   Normal conditions: Normally the heart and lungs play the main role for the circulation of qi and blood, but the liver has the ability to regulate and maintain the free flow of qi and blood in order to prevent the stagnation of qi and blood.
   Abnormal conditions: If the liver does not keep qi and blood flowing freely, the following unhealthy conditions could result: pain or distension in the breasts or upper rib area, painful or fixed mass in upper abdomen, abnormal menstruation (painful or absent), and more.

3. **Dominating and Controlling the Tendons and Manifesting in the Nails**

   In traditional Chinese medicine, the dominance and control of a zang organ means that the organ is vital for the flow of qi and blood for the associated body tissues. For example, the tendons and nails need nourishment from qi and blood. Liver blood will nourish the tendons and nails. Therefore, the liver is the key organ to dominate and control the functions of the tendons and nails.

   Normal conditions: Liver blood nourishes the tendons and maintains their normal function. The tendons link the joints and muscles and dominate and control the movement of the four extremities.

   Abnormal conditions: If the liver does not function well, it could cause malnutrition of the tendons, which could result in numbness of the extremities, slower movement of the joints, spasms, tremors in the hands and feet, and more. If liver blood is deficient or has poor quality, the nails could become soft, thin, and brittle.

4. **Opening into the Eyes through the Meridians**

   In traditional Chinese medicine, every zang organ has one function that opens into one sense organ. For the Wood element, the liver opens into the eyes. This means the liver's meridian connects with the eyes. In allopathic medicine the liver and eyes are completely separate organs. But they are connected through the meridians, which are the pathways of qi.

   Normal conditions: Liver blood nourishes the eyes to ensure normal eye function with clear vision.

   Abnormal conditions: Lack of liver blood could result in blurred vision, night blindness, and dry eyes.

Soul Healing for the Liver and Wood Element

Now I am formally releasing soul healing techniques for the liver. When we do soul healing for the liver (the zang organ of the Wood element), the gallbladder (the fu organ of the Wood element), the eyes (the sense organ), the tendons (the body tissue), and anger in the emotional body will all receive the healing simultaneously. To offer soul healing to the authority (zang) organ is to offer healing to everything connected with the Wood element.

Apply the Four Power Techniques:

Body Power. Place the right palm on the liver area. Place the left palm on the lower abdomen below the navel.

Soul Power. Say *hello* to inner souls:

> *Dear soul mind body of my liver, gallbladder, eyes, tendons, and the emotional body of the Wood element,*
> *I love you, honor you, and appreciate you.*
> *You have the power to heal and rejuvenate my liver, gallbladder, eyes, and tendons and to heal my anger.*
> *Do a good job!*
> *Thank you.*

Say *hello* to outer souls:

> *Dear Divine,*
> *Dear Tao, The Source,*
> *I love you, honor you, and appreciate you.*
> *Please forgive my ancestors and me for all the mistakes we have made in all lifetimes related to the liver, gallbladder, eyes, tendons, and anger.*
> *I am sincerely sorry for all of these mistakes.*
> *I apologize from the bottom of my heart to all the souls my ancestors and I have hurt or harmed in these ways.*
> *I apologize to you, dear Divine and Tao.*
> *In order to be forgiven, I will serve unconditionally.*
> *To chant and meditate is to serve.*
> *I will chant and meditate as much as I can.*
> *I will offer unconditional service as much as I can.*
> *I am extremely grateful.*
> *Thank you.*

Mind Power. Visualize bright green light shining in and around the liver. Bright green light has special healing power for the Wood element.

Sound Power. Chant silently or aloud as follows for at least ten minutes. The longer you practice, the better.

> *Liver regulates blood.*
> *Liver promotes qi and blood flow.*
> *Eyes are clear and bright.*
> *Tendons and nails are healthy.*
> *Anger is removed...*

I have bolded these chanting lines because this is the first time that I have released this sacred soul healing by chanting these phrases.

How does it work? Remember my teaching: *everything is made of soul, mind, and body*. Every system, organ, cell, and every DNA and RNA has a soul, mind, and body. They have the power to self-heal and rejuvenate. This kind of healing has not been offered in history or at least has not been offered enough. This is soul healing for the Five Elements' systems, organs, tissues, cells, meridians, acupuncture points, and the emotional body.

My foundation teaching of Soul Mind Body Medicine is *Heal the soul first; then healing of the mind and body will follow*. Soul is spirit, information, and message. To chant these bolded phrases is soul healing or message healing. It has power beyond words. I am honored and delighted to release soul healing by applying the ancient wisdom of the Five Elements to you and humanity. I wish for you to practice a lot and receive maximum healing benefits. I wish for you to create your own soul healing miracles.

Now I will lead you to apply all Four Power Techniques together with the fifth sacred technique of healing, Breath Power.

There are so many ways to breathe. I would like every reader to focus on one way to breathe. It is named abdominal breathing. When you inhale, your abdomen expands. When you exhale, your abdomen contracts. Make sure you inhale and exhale smoothly and evenly. The length of each inhale and exhale depends on your personal condition. It could be different for everyone. Follow nature's way. As you continue to practice in this way, the length of your inhale and exhale will get longer, little by little. The key principle is to *follow nature's way*. Remember never to purposely prolong your breathing. The length of your inhale and exhale will increase naturally through more practice.

I will now lead you through a breathing practice.

Sit up straight. Place the tip of your tongue gently against the roof of your mouth. Place one palm on the liver and place the other palm below the navel.

Inhale deeply. Your abdomen will expand. Put your mind on your liver. Then exhale. Put your mind on your whole body. Practice by inhaling and exhaling slowly ten times.

> Inhale, exhale
> Inhale, exhale
> Inhale, exhale
> Inhale, exhale...

The first step is to train your mind. Then we will add the chanting.

Relax. For ten minutes, inhale and expand the abdomen. Focus your mind on the liver and at the same time chant *Liver regulates blood*. Exhale and the abdomen contracts. Focus your mind on the whole body and at the same time chant *Da Ai* (pronounced *dah eye,* which means *greatest love*).

Let me explain the significance of this practice.

Inhaling and exhaling are a yin yang pair. This is Breath Power.

Focusing your mind on the liver and on the whole body is another yin yang pair. This is Mind Power.

Chanting *Liver regulates blood* and *Da Ai* is another yin yang pair. This is Sound Power.

Placing one hand over the liver and placing one hand on the lower abdomen is another yin yang pair. This is Body Power.

Invoking the Source, the Divine, and Heaven's countless spiritual fathers and mothers to bless your liver and body is another yin yang pair. This is Soul Power.

We have practiced the Four Power Techniques a lot in the last ten years in my Soul Power Series books and other books. These Four Power Techniques have created hundreds of thousands of soul healing miracles. We are very grateful for the Four Power Techniques. The Divine, Tao, and the ancient wisdom of my spiritual fathers and mothers guided me to create the Four Power Techniques.

Now we are going to add Breath Power, which is the fifth Power Technique, wherever and whenever it is appropriate.

I have explained that every power technique has yin and yang aspects. Why is the yin yang pair alternating practice sacred and vital? It can be summarized in one sentence:

> **Yin yang alternating practice is to balance yin and yang**
> **and to join yin and yang as One, which is to meld with Tao.**

One is Tao. Tao is One. Tao is The Way of all life, including healing, rejuvenation, prolonging life, and transforming relationships, finances, and more.

Now let us practice.

Breath Power, Mind Power, Sound Power, Soul Power, and Body Power (Five Power Techniques) Together

Sit up straight. Place the tip of your tongue gently against the roof of your mouth. Place one palm over your liver and place your other palm on the lower abdomen below the navel. Deeply inhale, keeping your mind on your liver by visualizing bright green light shining in and around the liver. Silently chant *Liver regulates blood well*.

When you exhale, put your mind on the whole body by visualizing bright green light radiating throughout the whole body. Silently chant *Da Ai* (pronounced *dah eye*) or *Greatest Love*.

Now do the practice for the second time.

Deeply inhale, keeping your mind on your liver, visualizing bright green light there. Silently chant *Liver regulates blood well*.

Exhale, putting your mind on your whole body, visualizing bright green light radiating throughout the whole body. Silently chant *Da Ai* or *Greatest Love*.

Stop reading and practice for two minutes.

Now let us move to the second sacred chant for healing the liver and everything associated with the Wood element, including the gallbladder, eyes, tendons, and anger in the emotional body.

Deeply inhale, keeping your mind on your liver. Silently chant *Liver promotes qi and blood flow*.

When you exhale, put your mind on your whole body. Silently chant *Da Kuan Shu* (pronounced *dah kwahn shoo*) or *Greatest Forgiveness*.

Chant and visualize for two minutes.

Next, deeply inhale, keeping your mind on your liver and silently chant *Tendons and nails are healthy*.

When you exhale, put your mind on your whole body and silently chant *Da Ci Bei* (pronounced *dah sz bay*) or *Greatest Compassion*.

Chant and visualize for another two minutes.

Then deeply inhale, keeping your mind on your liver and silently chant *Eyes are clear and bright*.

When you exhale, put your mind on the whole body and silently chant *Da Guang Ming* (pronounced *dah gwahng ming*) or *Greatest Light*.

Chant and visualize for another two minutes.

Now I will lead you to practice this sacred chanting as one. For healing the Wood element, including the liver, gallbladder, eyes, tendons, and anger in the emotional body, always visualize bright green light.

Deeply inhale, keeping your mind on your liver, and silently chant *Liver regulates blood well*.

Then exhale and silently chant *Da Ai* (pronounced *dah eye*) or *Greatest Love*, putting your mind on the whole body.

Then deeply inhale and silently chant *Liver promotes qi and blood flow*.

Then exhale and silently chant *Da Kuan Shu* (pronounced *dah kwahn shoo*) or *Greatest Forgiveness*.

Now, deeply inhale and silently chant *Tendons and nails are healthy*.

Exhale and silently chant *Da Ci Bei* (pronounced *dah sz bay*) or *Greatest Compassion*.

Continue to inhale deeply and silently chant *Eyes are clear and bright*.

Finally, exhale and silently chant *Da Guang Ming* (pronounced *dah gwahng ming*) or *Greatest Light*.

Now stop reading. Continue to chant and visualize for ten minutes. For chronic or life-threatening conditions of the liver, gallbladder, eyes, tendons, or anger, chant two hours or more per day. You can add up all of your chanting time to total at least two hours per day.

I emphasize again that this is the first time that I have released this sacred practice with the Five Power Techniques. The name of this new practice is *Sacred Yin Yang Alternation Practice*.

Heart

The heart lies in the left chest and is surrounded by the pericardium. The heart is the zang (authority) organ of the Fire element. The fu organ of the Fire element is the small intestine. The meridians of the heart and small intestine are internally and externally related.

1. **Governing the Blood and Blood Vessels**
   In traditional Chinese medicine, dominating, controlling, and governing have the same meaning. They are the key function of the heart.
   Normal conditions: The heart is the driving force for blood circulation in the whole body, and the blood vessels house and circulate the blood. A healthy heart includes adequate qi and blood, open blood vessels, and a regular, healthy, and strong heartbeat.
   Abnormal conditions: A lack of blood in the heart could manifest as a weak pulse, irregular heartbeat, and more.

2. **Manifesting on the Face**
   Normal conditions: If the heart has good circulation and the blood supply is sufficient to the face, the complexion could appear pink and glowing.
   Abnormal conditions: If heart circulation, blood supply, and pulse are poor, the complexion could appear pale. If heart circulation is stagnant, the face could appear blue or purple.

3. **Housing the Mind and Taking Charge of Mental Activities**
   Normal conditions: Traditional Chinese medicine emphasizes that the heart houses the mind and soul. The heart connects with the soul's activities, consciousness, and thinking. If the heart and

blood circulation function perfectly, the mental outlook is positive, energetic, and healthy.

Abnormal conditions: An imbalance in the function of the heart and blood circulation could result in mental disorder, insomnia, palpitations, dream-disturbed sleep, and more.

4. **Opening into the Tongue through the Meridians**
   Normal conditions: The heart is the governing organ for the sense of taste. The tongue should appear moist, pink, and shiny, have a normal sense of taste, and be able to move freely.
   Abnormal conditions: An incomplete supply of heart blood could result in a pale, red, dark, or purple tongue. If the heart does not control mental activities well, the tongue may appear rigid, and confusion and an inability to speak could occur.

5. **Sweat Is the Fluid of the Heart**
   Normal conditions: Traditional Chinese medicine states that blood and sweat come from the same source. Normal perspiration is a sign of a healthy heart and blood circulation.
   Abnormal conditions: Excessive perspiration could result in palpitations, accelerated heartbeat, loss of bodily fluid, and more.

Now let us do a few minutes of practice for soul healing the heart. If you have circulation or other heart issues, this practice will offer you healing. If you do not have circulation or heart issues, always remember that the practice can still benefit you by strengthening the heart, preventing heart sickness, and rejuvenating the heart. Every reader can benefit from this practice.

Sacred Yin Yang Alternation Practice for the Heart and Fire Element
Apply the Five Power Techniques together:

Body Power. Sit up straight. Place the tip of your tongue gently against the roof of your mouth. Place one palm over your heart. Place the other palm on your lower abdomen below the navel.

Soul Power. Say *hello* to inner souls:

> *Dear soul mind body of my heart, small intestine, tongue, blood*
>   *vessels, and emotional body of the Fire element,*
> *I love you, honor you, and appreciate you.*
> *You have the power to heal and rejuvenate my heart, small intestine,*
>   *tongue, and blood vessels, which include the big and small arteries,*
>   *capillaries, and small and big veins, and to heal depression and anxiety.*
> *Do a good job!*
> *Thank you.*

 Say *hello* to outer souls:

> *Dear Divine,*
> *Dear Tao, The Source,*
> *I love you, honor you, and appreciate you.*
> *Please forgive my ancestors and me for all the mistakes we have*
>   *made in all lifetimes related to the heart, small intestine, tongue,*
>   *blood vessels, capillary system, and depression and anxiety.*
> *In order to be forgiven, I will serve unconditionally.*
> *To chant and meditate is to serve.*
> *I will chant and meditate as much as I can.*
> *I will offer unconditional service as much as I can.*
> *I am extremely grateful.*
> *Thank you.*

Mind Power. Visualize bright red light shining in the heart area. Bright red light has special healing power for the Fire element.

Sound Power. Chant silently or aloud:

> *Heart circulates perfectly.*
> *Complexion is glowing.*
> *Clear mind.*
> *Perfect tongue.*
> *Normal perspiration…*

When you do the practice for healing the heart and Fire element, always remember to visualize bright red light in the heart as you inhale, and bright *golden* light throughout the body as you exhale.

Now inhale deeply, keeping your mind on your heart by visualizing bright red light shining in your heart. Silently chant *Heart circulates perfectly*.

Exhale and put your mind on your whole body by visualizing bright golden light. Silently chant *Da Ai* (pronounced *dah eye*) or *Greatest Love*.

Inhale deeply, keeping your mind on your heart by visualizing bright red light. Silently chant *Complexion is glowing. Perfect tongue*.

Exhale and put your mind on your whole body by visualizing bright golden light. Silently chant *Da Kuan Shu* (pronounced *dah kwahn shoo*) or *Greatest Forgiveness*.

Inhale deeply, keeping your mind on your heart (red light). Silently chant *Clear mind*.

Exhale and put your mind on your whole body (golden light). Silently chant *Da Ci Bei* (pronounced *dah sz bay*) or *Greatest Compassion*.

Then inhale deeply, keeping your mind on your heart. Silently chant *Normal perspiration*.

Finally, exhale and put your mind on your whole body and silently chant *Da Guang Ming* (pronounced *dah gwahng ming*) or *Greatest Light*.

Now stop reading. Continue to chant and visualize for ten minutes. For chronic or life-threatening conditions, chant two hours or more per day. You can add up all of your chanting time to total at least two hours per day.

Spleen

The spleen is located in the Middle Jiao, in the left upper abdomen, to the left of the stomach. In traditional Chinese medicine, the spleen is the zang (authority) organ of the Earth element, which is in charge of the digestive system. The fu organ of the Earth element is the stomach. The meridians of the spleen and stomach are internally and externally related.

1. **Absorbing, Transporting, Distributing, and Transforming Nutrients in Order to Nourish the Whole Body, from Head to Toe, Skin to Bone**
   This function of the spleen includes two aspects:

a) Absorbing, Distributing, and Transforming Nutrients

Traditional Chinese medicine teaches that food and water travel to the stomach. The stomach and spleen digest and transform the food. The essence of the food is sent by the spleen's function up to the lungs. From there, the lungs spread the food essence to the whole body to nourish the five zang and six fu organs along with the four extremities, bones, skin, and hair. Water and the essence of food are the materials to form blood. Therefore, the spleen is the root organ to produce qi (energy) and blood after birth.

Normal conditions: A healthy spleen is the key for producing qi and blood for the whole body. The spleen is also the key organ to transport, distribute, transform, and absorb food essence and water.

Abnormal conditions: Difficulties in transporting, distributing, and transforming food could result in poor appetite, indigestion, issues with the bowels, weight loss, and more. Difficulties in absorbing and transporting water could result in diarrhea, water retention, edema, and more.

b) Transporting and Transforming Liquids

Normal conditions: Traditional Chinese medicine teaches that the spleen is the main zang organ to transport and transform liquids and secretions in the body. The spleen transports the liquids to the lungs and the liquids are divided into clear and unclear. The clear liquids nourish the five zang organs and the six fu organs internally. The unclear liquids are further transformed to perspiration, urine, or stool and excreted externally.

Abnormal conditions: If there are blockages in the transportation and transformation of liquids, one could experience edema, phlegm retention, diarrhea, and more.

2. **Controlling and Maintaining Blood Flow within the Blood Vessels**

Normal conditions: Spleen qi (energy) has the power to keep the blood flowing within the blood vessels. A healthy spleen produces strong spleen qi and strong blood, and will ensure that blood flows within the blood vessels.

Abnormal conditions: If the spleen has an insufficient supply of qi, blood in the stool and urine, hemorrhaging, and more could result.

3. **Dominating the Muscles and Four Extremities**
    Normal conditions: The spleen has the power to nourish the muscles. If the spleen functions normally and nutrients are distributed well throughout the body, the muscles and extremities are strong and well-developed.
    Abnormal conditions: If spleen qi is weak or depleted, the muscles and extremities could become weak and loose.

4. **Opening into the Mouth through the Meridians and Manifesting on the Lips**
    Normal conditions: A healthy spleen manifests a healthy appetite, a normal sense of taste, and pink lips.
    Abnormal conditions: Stagnant qi within the spleen could result in poor appetite, a diminished sense of taste, a feeling of fullness in the upper abdomen, and more.

Sacred Yin Yang Alternation Practice for the Spleen and Earth Element
Apply the Five Power Techniques together:

Body Power. Sit up straight. Place the tip of your tongue gently against the roof of your mouth. Place one palm over your spleen. Place your other palm on your lower abdomen below the navel.

Soul Power. Say *hello* to inner souls:

> *Dear soul mind body of my spleen, stomach, muscles, mouth, lips,*
>   *teeth, gums, and emotional body of the Earth element,*
> *I love you, honor you, and appreciate you.*
> *You have the power to heal and rejuvenate my spleen, stomach,*
>   *muscles, mouth, lips, teeth, and gums and to heal worry.*
> *Do a good job!*
> *Thank you.*

Say *hello* to outer souls:

> *Dear Divine,*
> *Dear Tao, The Source,*
> *I love you, honor you, and appreciate you.*
> *Please forgive my ancestors and me for all the mistakes we have*
>   *made in all lifetimes related to the spleen, stomach, muscles,*
>   *mouth, lips, teeth, gums, and worry.*
> *I am sincerely sorry for all of these mistakes.*
> *In order to be forgiven, I will serve unconditionally.*
> *To chant and meditate is to serve.*
> *I will chant and meditate as much as I can.*
> *I will offer unconditional service as much as I can.*
> *I am extremely grateful.*
> *Thank you.*

Mind Power. Visualize bright golden light shining in and around the spleen. Bright golden light has special healing power for the Earth element.

Sound Power. Chant silently or aloud:

> *Absorb food essence and water.*
> *Strengthen spleen qi.*
> *Strong muscles and limbs.*
> *Perfect mouth, lips, gums, and teeth…*

When you do the practice for healing the spleen and Earth element, always remember to visualize bright golden light in the spleen and throughout the body as you inhale and exhale.

Now inhale deeply, keeping your mind on your spleen by visualizing bright golden light shining in and around your spleen. Silently chant *Absorb food essence and water*.

Now exhale and put your mind on your whole body by visualizing bright golden light. Silently chant *Da Ai* (pronounced *dah eye*) or *Greatest Love*.

Inhale deeply, keeping your mind on your spleen. Silently chant *Strengthen spleen qi*.

Exhale and put your mind on your whole body, visualizing bright golden light. Silently chant *Da Kuan Shu* (pronounced *dah kwahn shoo*) or *Greatest Forgiveness*.

Inhale deeply, keeping your mind on your spleen. Silently chant *Strong muscles and limbs*.

Exhale and put your mind on your whole body. Silently chant *Da Ci Bei* (pronounced *dah sz bay*) or *Greatest Compassion*.

Then inhale deeply, keeping your mind on your spleen. Silently chant *Perfect mouth, lips, gums, and teeth*.

Finally, exhale and put your mind on your whole body and silently chant *Da Guang Ming* (pronounced *dah gwahng ming*), or *Greatest Light*.

Now stop reading. Continue to chant and visualize for ten minutes. For chronic or life-threatening conditions, chant two hours or more per day. You can add up all of your chanting time to total at least two hours per day.

Lungs

The lungs are located in the thoracic cavity of the chest, with one lung on the right and one on the left. The lungs are the zang (authority) organ of the Metal element. The fu organ of the Metal element is the large intestine. The meridians of the lungs and large intestine are internally and externally related.

1. **Dominating Qi, including Respiratory Qi and Whole Body Qi**
   a) **Controlling the Qi of Respiration**
   Normal conditions: The lungs are the primary organ for the internal intake of oxygen and the external release of carbon dioxide. This allows the body's metabolism to function smoothly. Respiration remains normal and smooth if there are no obstructions in the main qi of the lungs.
   Abnormal conditions: A deficiency of lung qi could lead to respiratory disorders, breathing difficulties, asthma, coughing, fatigue, and more.

b) Controlling the Qi of the Whole Body
Normal conditions: The lungs help to form zong qi ("gathering qi," pronounced *dzawng chee*). Zong qi is formed by fresh air inhaled by the lungs together with the food essence sent by the spleen. Zong qi is sent up by the spleen to the larynx, where it gathers to influence speech and give strength to the voice. It promotes the function of the lungs and nourishes all organs, systems, tissues, and every part of the body.
Abnormal conditions: If this function of the lungs is weak, the formation of zong qi could be affected. Shortness of breath, a weak voice, fatigue, exhaustion, and more could result.

2. **Dominating, Descending, and Distributing Qi, Food Essence, and Body Fluids to All Systems, Organs, and Meridians, as Well as Skin, Hair, and Muscles**
Normal conditions: The lungs distribute the food essence and body fluids throughout the whole body in order to nourish the whole body. Lung qi normally flows downward. The lungs are also the principal organ to nourish the skin and hair. The pores of the skin are the openings for qi. If the Upper Jiao is healthy, functions properly, and transports the proper amounts of high-quality qi, body fluids, and nutrients, then the skin and whole body are nourished and the hair and muscles are healthy.
Abnormal conditions: If the qi in the lungs cannot flow downward, coughing, asthma, fullness in the chest, and more could result. If the lungs lack high-quality qi, the skin could appear sallow, pale, and dry.

3. **Regulating the Water Passages and Helping to Maintain Normal Water Metabolism**
Normal conditions: The lungs have the function of transporting liquid to the kidneys and urinary bladder. Then there is easy elimination of urine. This allows for normal water metabolism.
Abnormal conditions: If there is dysfunction of the lung qi and imbalance of water metabolism, edema, lack of urine, painful urination, and more could result.

4. **Opening into the Nose through the Meridians**
   Normal conditions: The nose is the pathway for inhaling and exhaling air. If the nose has no obstructions and high-quality qi, the nose will develop a powerful sense of smell.
   Abnormal conditions: If qi is obstructed within the nose, a stuffy nose, runny nose, impaired sense of smell, and more could result.

Sacred Yin Yang Alternation Practice for the Lungs and Metal Element

Apply the Five Power Techniques together:

Body Power. Sit up straight. Place the tip of your tongue gently against the roof of your mouth. Place one hand over one or both lungs. Place your other hand on your lower abdomen below the navel.

Soul Power. Say *hello* to inner souls:

> *Dear soul mind body of my lungs, large intestine, skin, nose, and*
> *emotional body of the Metal element,*
> *I love you, honor you, and appreciate you.*
> *You have the power to heal and rejuvenate my lungs, large intestine,*
> *skin, and nose and to heal grief.*
> *Do a good job!*
> *Thank you.*

Say *hello* to outer souls:

> *Dear Divine,*
> *Dear Tao, The Source,*
> *I love you, honor you, and appreciate you.*
> *Please forgive my ancestors and me for all the mistakes we have*
> *made in all lifetimes related to the lungs, large intestine, skin,*
> *nose, and grief.*
> *I am deeply sorry from the bottom of my heart for all of these*
> *mistakes.*
> *In order to be forgiven, I will serve unconditionally.*

To chant and meditate is to serve.
I will chant and meditate as much as I can.
I will offer unconditional service as much as I can.
I am extremely grateful.
Thank you.

Mind Power. Visualize bright white light shining in and around your lungs. Bright white light has special healing power for the Metal element.

Sound Power. Chant silently or aloud:

Powerful qi.
Food essence and liquids nourish whole body.
Perfect metabolism.
Normal nose functions…

When you do the practice for healing the lungs and Metal element, always remember to visualize bright white light in the lungs and throughout the body as you inhale and exhale.

Now inhale deeply, keeping your mind on your lungs by visualizing bright white light shining in your lungs. Silently chant *Powerful qi.*

Now exhale and put your mind on your whole body by visualizing bright white light. Silently chant *Da Ai* (pronounced *dah eye*) or *Greatest Love.*

Inhale deeply, keeping your mind on your lungs (white light). Silently chant *Food essence and liquids nourish whole body.*

Exhale and put your mind on your whole body, visualizing bright white light. Silently chant *Da Kuan Shu* (pronounced *dah kwahn shoo*) or *Greatest Forgiveness.*

Inhale deeply, keeping your mind on your lungs. Silently chant *Perfect metabolism.*

Exhale and put your mind on your whole body and silently chant *Da Ci Bei* (pronounced *dah sz bay*) or *Greatest Compassion.*

Then inhale deeply, keeping your mind on your lungs. Silently chant *Normal nose functions.*

Finally, exhale and put your mind on your whole body and silently chant *Da Guang Ming* (pronounced *dah gwahng ming*) or *Greatest Light*.

Now stop reading. Continue to chant and visualize for ten minutes. For chronic or life-threatening conditions, chant two hours or more per day. You can add up all of your chanting time to total at least two hours per day.

Kidneys

The kidneys are located in the loins on either side of the spinal column.

The kidneys are the zang (authority) organ of the Water element. The fu organ of the Water element is the urinary bladder. The meridians of the kidneys and urinary bladder are internally and externally related.

1. **Storing Pre-natal and Post-natal Jing (Matter) and Dominating Development and Reproduction**

   a) **Inherited Essence of Life**
   Normal conditions: The vital inherited essence of life is stored within the kidneys both before and after birth. It is inherited from the mother and father and then developed by the nutrients and other essences taken into the body. This vital inherited essence of life is then transformed into qi to assist the body to grow, develop, and reproduce.
   Abnormal conditions: If there is a lack of essential nutrients and vital qi through development and reproduction, as well as an imbalance of yin yang, slow development, premature senility, hot flashes, coldness in the hands and feet, infertility, impotence, and more could result.

   b) **Developed Essence of Life**
   Normal conditions: The developed essence of life is held and used by the five zang organs and the six fu organs. It is derived from food essence. The food essence is transformed by the spleen and stomach into this developed essence of life and then transported to the five zang organs and the six fu organs. When this developed essence of life is sufficient, any excess is stored in the kidneys for future use.

Abnormal conditions: If at any time the developed essence of life in the five zang organs and six fu organs is insufficient, the kidneys will send their stored essence to the five zang organs and six fu organs. Sensations of heat in the chest, palms, and soles of the feet, night sweats, cold and pain in the lumbar spine area and knees, infertility, frigidity, and more could result.

2. **Dominating Water Metabolism**
   Normal conditions: Normal functioning of the kidneys maintains the proper balance of fluids and sustains water circulation in the body. Body fluid carries a valuable nourishing purpose that has come from the food essence. It is distributed to the five zang organs, the six fu organs, and the tissues throughout the body. Proper urination occurs with healthy water metabolism.
   Abnormal conditions: If there are blockages in healthy water metabolism and water circulation, edema, frequent or infrequent urination, and more can result.

3. **Receiving Qi**
   Normal conditions: Traditional Chinese medicine teaches that the kidneys support the lungs in the inhaling of air downwards. Kidney qi must be strong for the lungs to inhale and exhale easily.
   Abnormal conditions: If kidney qi has any weakness, breathing difficulties could result.

4. **Dominating the Bones, Manufacturing Marrow to Fill the Brain, and Manifesting in the Hair**
   Normal conditions: The kidneys store the essence of life, which is then transformed into bone marrow. When the kidney qi is substantial enough, high-quality bone marrow is produced, leading to healthy and firm bones and teeth. The hair is nourished by the blood and is the external manifestation of the kidneys. The hair will then appear shiny and healthy.
   Abnormal conditions: A lack of kidney qi could result in insufficient nourishment for the bones. Weakness and soreness in the back and weakness in the feet and knees could then develop.

The bones could become brittle and weak. This could also lead to loose teeth or the loss of teeth, baldness, gray hair, and more.

5. **Opening into the Ears through the Meridians and Dominating Anterior and Posterior Orifices**
   Normal conditions: If the kidneys receive the appropriate amount of nourishment or qi, one could have very clear hearing and proper elimination.
   Abnormal conditions: If kidney qi is insufficient, tinnitus (ringing in the ears), loss of hearing or sensitivity to sound, diarrhea, constipation, impotence, infertility, frequent urination, and more could result.

Sacred Yin Yang Alternation Practice for the Kidneys and Water Element
Apply the Five Power Techniques together:

Body Power. Sit up straight. Place the tip of your tongue gently against the roof of your mouth. Place one palm over a kidney. Place your other palm on your lower abdomen below the navel.

Soul Power. Say *hello* to inner souls:

> *Dear soul mind body of my kidneys, urinary bladder, bones, ears,*
>   *and emotional body of the Water element,*
> *I love you, honor you, and appreciate you.*
> *You have the power to heal and rejuvenate my kidneys, urinary*
>   *bladder, bones, and ears and to heal fear.*
> *Do a good job!*
> *Thank you.*

Say *hello* to outer souls:

> *Dear Divine,*
> *Dear Tao, The Source,*
> *I love you, honor you, and appreciate you.*

Please forgive my ancestors and me for all the mistakes we have
    made in all lifetimes related to the kidneys, urinary bladder,
    bones, ears, and fear.
I am sincerely sorry for all of these mistakes.
I apologize from the bottom of my heart to all the souls my ancestors
    and I have hurt or harmed in these ways.
In order to be forgiven, I will serve unconditionally.
To chant and meditate is to serve.
I will chant and meditate as much as I can.
I will offer unconditional service as much as I can.
I am extremely grateful.
Thank you.

Mind Power. Visualize bright blue light shining in and around the kidneys. Bright blue light has special healing power for the Water element.

Sound Power. Chant silently or aloud:

    Strong kidney jing and qi.
    Normal water metabolism.
    Strong bones, bone marrow, and healthy hair.
    Clear hearing and normal elimination…

When you do the practice for healing the kidneys and Water element, always remember to visualize bright blue light in the kidneys and throughout the body as you inhale and exhale.

Now inhale deeply, keeping your mind on your kidneys by visualizing bright blue light shining in and around your kidneys. Silently chant *Strong kidney jing and qi.*

Now exhale and put your mind on your whole body by visualizing bright blue light. Silently chant *Da Ai* (pronounced *dah eye*) or *Greatest Love.*

Inhale deeply, keeping your mind on your kidneys. Silently chant *Normal water metabolism.*

Exhale and put your mind on your whole body, visualizing bright blue light. Silently chant *Da Kuan Shu* (pronounced *dah kwahn shoo)* or *Greatest Forgiveness.*

Inhale deeply, keeping your mind on your kidneys. Silently chant *Strong bones, bone marrow, and healthy hair.*

Exhale and put your mind on your whole body. Silently chant *Da Ci Bei* (pronounced *dah sz bay)* or *Greatest Compassion.*

Then inhale deeply, keeping your mind on your kidneys. Silently chant *Clear hearing and normal elimination.*

Finally, exhale, putting your mind on your whole body and silently chant *Da Guang Ming* (pronounced *dah gwahng ming)* or *Greatest Light.*

Now stop reading. Continue to chant and visualize for ten minutes. For chronic or life-threatening conditions, chant two hours or more per day. You can add up all of your chanting time to total at least two hours per day.

In this chapter we have done soul healing for each of the authority organs of the Five Elements: liver, heart, spleen, lungs, and kidneys. When you do these soul healing practices, healing is automatically offered to the six fu organs and more.

Healing the Five Zang Organs, Six Fu Organs, and Extraordinary Organs Together

Now I am delighted to release the sacred wisdom, knowledge, and practical techniques for soul healing all organs, all systems, all tissues, and all sense organs of the Five Elements together, along with the emotional body and the extraordinary organs (brain, bone marrow, bones, and uterus).

Apply the Five Power Techniques:

Body Power. Sit up straight with your back free and clear. Place your hands in the Five Elements Hand Position or Five Elements Hands Shen Mi by taking your left hand and placing all of the fingers together. Grasp the fingers of your left hand with your right hand. Place both hands on the lower abdomen below the navel. See figure 7.

In using the Five Elements Hands Shen Mi (Body Secret), a further secret is to alternate your grip between very strong and very gentle. Grip your left fingers hard for about thirty seconds. Then grip your fingers with hardly any strength for thirty seconds. Keep alternating yang and yin in this way.

Let me explain the sacred healing.

The index finger connects with the Wood element, including the liver, gallbladder, tendons, eyes, anger in the emotional body, and more.

The middle finger connects with the Fire element, including the heart, small intestine, blood vessels, tongue, depression and anxiety in the emotional body, and more.

The ring finger connects with the Metal element, including the lungs, large intestine, skin, nose, grief in the emotional body, and more.

The baby finger connects with the Water element, including the kidneys, urinary bladder, bones, ears, fear in the emotional body, and more.

The thumb connects with the Earth element, including the spleen, stomach, muscles, mouth, lips, gums, teeth, worry in the emotional body, and more.

All of these connections are through the meridians. The meridians are the pathways of energy. This sacred healing has power beyond words.

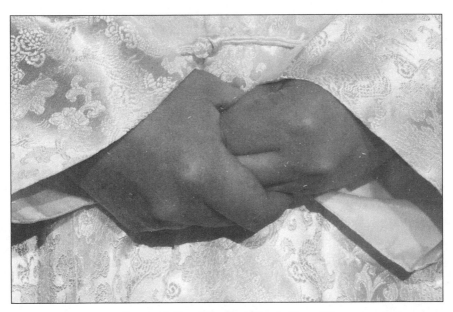

FIGURE 7. Five Elements Hands Shen Mi

Soul Power. Say *hello*:

> *Dear Divine,*
> *Dear Tao, The Source,*
> *Dear Five Elements,*
> *I love you, honor you, and appreciate you.*
> *Please forgive my ancestors and me for all the mistakes we have*
>   *made in all lifetimes related to the five zang organs, six fu organs,*
>   *four extremities, skin, hair, bones, and the emotional body.*
> *In order to be forgiven, I will serve humanity and all souls of Mother*
>   *Earth unconditionally.*
> *I will chant and meditate a lot to bring unconditional love,*
>   *forgiveness, compassion, and light to humanity, Mother Earth, and*
>   *all universes.*
> *Thank you.*

Sound Power. Chant silently or aloud:

> *Wu Xing He Yi* (pronounced *woo shing huh yee*)

"Wu Xing" means *Five Elements.* "He Yi" means *join as one.* "Wu Xing He Yi" (pronounced *woo shing huh yee*) means *Five Elements join as one.*

Traditional Chinese medicine has much wisdom and many practices and applications for each element. Doctors of traditional Chinese medicine will diagnose and offer herbs, acupuncture, or Chinese massage as treatment. Five Elements theory and practice has served billions of people in history. I cannot honor traditional Chinese medicine enough. I cannot honor enough the scholars of five thousand years ago who discovered and offered the wisdom and practices of the Five Elements.

Now I am releasing a soul healing secret. Let me explain how this sacred soul healing works.

According to Soul Mind Body Medicine, every system, every organ, every cell, and every DNA and RNA is made of jing qi shen. Every sickness is due to the blockages of jing qi shen. To remove these blockages is to heal.

If the jing qi shen of the systems, organs, and cells of the Five Elements join as one, the person is healthy, energized, rejuvenated, and harmonized. All sickness can be explained as the jing qi shen of the systems, organs, and cells of the Five Elements *not* joining as one. Therefore, to join the Five Elements as one *is* sacred soul healing. This healing is beyond any imagination.

Let me lead you to practice. You will understand the power.

Apply the Five Power Techniques. Combine Body Power, Soul Power, Sound Power, Breath Power, and Mind Power together:

Breath Power and Sound Power. Inhale and chant *Wu Xing He Yi* (pronounced *woo shing huh yee*) or *Five Elements join as one*.

Exhale and chant *Da Ai* (pronounced *dah eye*) or *Greatest Love*.

Inhale and chant *Wu Xing He Yi* or *Five Elements join as one*.

Exhale and chant *Da Kuan Shu* (pronounced *dah kwahn shoo*) or *Greatest Forgiveness*.

Inhale and chant *Wu Xing He Yi* or *Five Elements join as one*.

Exhale and chant *Da Ci Bei* (pronounced *dah sz bay*) or *Greatest Compassion*.

Inhale and chant *Wu Xing He Yi* or *Five Elements join as one*.

Exhale and chant *Da Guang Ming* (pronounced *dah gwahng ming*) or *Greatest Light*.

Keep the same hand position.

Chant:

Wu Xing He Yi, Da Ai
Wu Xing He Yi, Da Kuan Shu
Wu Xing He Yi, Da Ci Bei
Wu Xing He Yi, Da Guang Ming
Wu Xing He Yi, Da Ai, Greatest Love
Wu Xing He Yi, Da Kuan Shu, Greatest Forgiveness
Wu Xing He Yi, Da Ci Bei, Greatest Compassion
Wu Xing He Yi, Da Guang Ming, Greatest Light…

Five Elements join as one.
Five Elements join as one.
Five Elements join as one.
Five Elements join as one.
Five Elements join as one.
Five Elements join as one.
Five Elements join as one . . .

Mind Power. Inhale and put your mind on the Ming Men acupuncture point on the back directly behind the navel. See figure 8. See it as a bright golden light point. Exhale and visualize the whole body shining rainbow light from head to toe, skin to bone.

Stop reading now. Chant *Wu Xing He Yi* (pronounced *woo shing huh yee*), *Da Ai* (pronounced *dah eye*), *Greatest Love; Wu Xing He Yi, Da Kuan Shu* (pronounced *dah kwahn shoo*), *Greatest Forgiveness; Wu Xing He Yi, Da Ci Bei* (pronounced *dah sz bay*), *Greatest Compassion; Wu Xing He Yi, Da Guang Ming* (pronounced *dah gwahng ming*), *Greatest Light; and Five Elements join as one* for ten minutes and visualize at the same time.

I am delighted to emphasize again that this is one of the most profound sacred practices for soul healing.

Practice much more. This practice is for healing from head to toe, skin to bone, including the spiritual, mental, emotional, and physical bodies. There is no time limit to chanting and practicing. The more you chant and practice, the better. You can chant during your meditation. You can chant while cooking. You can chant while walking. You can chant during a break at work.

If you want to know if a pear is sweet, taste it. If you want to know if Wu Xing He Yi is powerful, experience it.

Practice. Practice. Practice.

I wish for you to create your own soul healing miracles. Share this sacred and simple wisdom and these practical techniques with your loved ones and humanity.

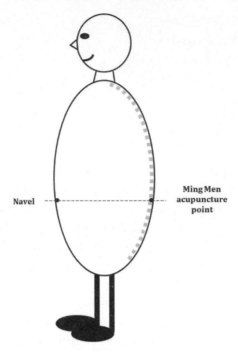

F<small>IGURE</small> 8. Ming Men acupuncture point

San Jiao (Pathway of Qi and Body Fluid)
and Wai Jiao (Biggest Space Inside the Body)

San Jiao is an important term and concept of traditional Chinese medicine. "San Jiao" (pronounced *sahn jee-yow*) means *three areas of the body: Upper Jiao, Middle Jiao*, and *Lower Jiao*. Upper Jiao is the area above the diaphragm, and includes the heart and lungs. Middle Jiao is the area between the diaphragm and the level of the navel, and includes the spleen and stomach. Lower Jiao is the area below the level of the navel to the genitals, and includes the liver, kidneys, urinary bladder, small and large intestines, and reproductive and sexual organs.

The main function of the Upper Jiao is to be in charge of respiration and blood circulation, as well as to spread jing and qi from food to nourish the whole body.

The main function of the Middle Jiao is to digest and absorb food, as well as to transform food to blood.

The main function of the Lower Jiao is to keep the essence of food and to eliminate urine and stool.

San Jiao is the pathway of qi and blood. To promote San Jiao flow is to promote qi and blood flow in the whole body. In chapter 5 you will learn how to apply the San Jiao to heal the whole body.

The Wai Jiao (pronounced *wye jee-yow*) is the biggest space in the body. It is located in front of the spinal column in the thoracic and abdominal cavities. See figure 9. The Wai Jiao was discovered in China by my spiritual mentor and father, Dr. and Master Zhi Chen Guo, after nearly fifty years of clinical research and practice with thousands of patients. He said, "San Jiao is like a river. Wai Jiao is like the ocean. The water from the river will flow to the ocean. Therefore, the blockages of the San Jiao move to the Wai Jiao. To clear the Wai Jiao is the key for healing."

There are so many ancient spiritual and energy wisdoms and practices for healing. There are also many sacred wisdoms and practices from traditional Chinese medicine, other types of medicine, and all kinds of healing modalities. I have shared a few important ancient wisdom secrets to help you understand spiritual and energy healing deeper and better. These ancient wisdoms and practices have served humanity and all souls for more than five thousand years. They will continue to serve more. Ancient secrets, wisdom, knowledge, and practical techniques have been proven through history to be extremely powerful. They will continue to empower humanity for healing and life transformation.

The Most Important Energy Circle and Matter Circle

In traditional Chinese medicine there are twelve regular meridians. Meridians are the pathways of energy. Every major organ has a meridian. Every meridian is important. What is the most important energy channel for the whole body?

On May 8, 2008, in my regular early-morning meditation, the Divine told me:

Dear Zhi Gang,
Today I am going to give you my fourth major Soul Song, the Divine Soul Song of Yin Yang. *This is my healing treasure for humanity.*

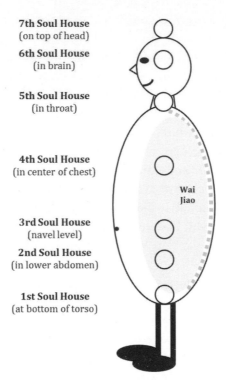

7th Soul House
(on top of head)

6th Soul House
(in brain)

5th Soul House
(in throat)

4th Soul House
(in center of chest)

Wai
Jiao

3rd Soul House
(navel level)

2nd Soul House
(in lower abdomen)

1st Soul House
(at bottom of torso)

FIGURE 9. Seven Soul Houses and Wai Jiao

I replied, "Thank you, Divine. I am extremely honored to receive your *Divine Soul Song of Yin Yang*. I understand how powerful this Divine Soul Song must be. To balance yin and yang is to heal all sicknesses."

The Divine said:

You are right. To balance yin and yang is the major healing principle in history. My Divine Soul Song of Yin Yang could help everyone balance their yin and yang. This is my healing treasure to empower people to heal themselves. You have been teaching self-healing for more than twenty years as I guided you to do. This Divine Soul Song is another step. Everyone can receive further benefits from it.

I replied, "Thank you so much. I am extremely honored to receive this priceless treasure."

The Divine continued:

Let me teach you about my Divine Soul Song of Yin Yang. *There are seven houses of the soul in a human being.*[5] *They are located in the center of the body* (see figure 9). *From lowest to highest, they are:*

- First Soul House—*just above the perineum, which is the region between the genitals and the anus*
- Second Soul House—*in the lower abdomen between the first Soul House and the level of the navel*
- Third Soul House—*at the level of the navel*
- Fourth Soul House—*the Message Center or heart chakra behind the sternum*
- Fifth Soul House—*in the throat*
- Sixth Soul House—*in the brain*
- Seventh Soul House—*the crown chakra on the top of the head*

There is also one area as you know named the Wai Jiao, which is the space in front of the spinal column. It is the biggest space in the body. From the first Soul House, move up to the second Soul House, then through the third, fourth, fifth, sixth, and seventh Soul Houses. Then turn down through the Wai Jiao back to the first Soul House. (See figure 10.)

I replied, "Dear Divine, thank you so much for the teaching. I understand that you are showing me the key energy circle for the whole body. I am very grateful and honored. I do have one question. In traditional Chinese medicine, the Ren meridian flows through the front midline of the body to the top of the head. The Du meridian flows through the back midline within the spinal cord to the top of the head. The Ren and Du meridians connect to form a vertical energy circle, which is itself a yin yang circle. You are teaching me to go up the middle of the body through the seven Soul Houses and then to go down through the Wai

---

[5] A human being lives in a house. Your beloved soul lives in your body. Your body is the house for your soul. There are seven Soul Houses where the soul can reside, which correspond to the chakras: at the bottom of the torso, in the lower abdomen, at the navel, in the center of the chest, in the throat, inside the brain, and on top of the head.

Jiao in front of the spinal column. How is this yin yang energy circle different from the Ren-Du meridian circle?"

The Divine replied:

The circle of the Ren-Du meridians is the yin yang circle in traditional Chinese Medicine and in Taoist practice. It is the Outer Yin Yang Circle. The circle I am showing you now is the Inner Yin Yang Circle. **The Inner Yin Yang Circle directs the Outer Yin Yang Circle.** *This is the greatest secret to balancing yin and yang in the body.*

I bowed down to the Divine 108 times to thank the Divine for revealing this divine secret to me to share with humanity. Then the Divine showed me the Soul Song for the entire energy circle.

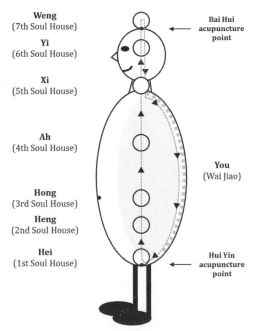

Hei Heng Hong Ah Xi Yi Weng You
(pronounced *hay hung hawng ah shee yee wung yoe*)

FIGURE 10. Most important energy circle in the body

The Divine said:

Hei Heng Hong Ah Xi Yi Weng You *forms the most important energy circle in the body. Every sickness is caused by blockages in soul, mind, and body. Soul blockages are bad karma. Mind blockages are blockages in consciousness, including negative mind-sets, negative attitudes, negative beliefs, ego, attachments, and more. Body blockages are energy and matter blockages. Blockages in soul, mind, and body will appear as blockages in this circle. To promote free flow of energy in this circle is to remove all blockages in soul, mind, and body. This circle is the Inner Yin Yang Circle.*

I am teaching you this so that you can share this teaching with humanity.

I bowed down again to show my gratitude to the Divine. I am so honored to share this wisdom with humanity.

Now let us do the practice. Choose one area for healing in the physical body, emotional body, mental body, or spiritual body.

Apply the Four Power Techniques:

Body Power. Sit up straight. Place the tip of your tongue gently against the roof of your mouth. Place one palm over the navel. Place the other palm over the Ming Men Acupuncture point directly behind the navel (figure 8).

Soul Power. Say *hello* to inner souls:

> *Dear soul mind body of my seven Soul Houses or seven energy chakras,*
> *Dear soul mind body of my Wai Jiao,*
> *I love you, honor you, and appreciate you.*
> *You have the power to heal all sicknesses.*
> *Please do a great job.*
> *Thank you.*

Say *hello* to outer souls:

> *Dear Divine,*
> *Dear Tao, The Source,*

Dear countless healing angels, archangels, ascended masters, gurus,
  lamas, kahunas, holy saints, Taoist saints, other saints, buddhas,
  bodhisattvas, and all kinds of spiritual fathers and mothers,
I love you, honor you, and appreciate you.
Please forgive my ancestors and me for all the mistakes we have
  made in all lifetimes,
In order to be forgiven, I will serve unconditionally.
To chant and to meditate is one of the greatest services.
I will chant and meditate more.
I also will do other acts of kindness for humanity.
Thank you. Thank you. Thank you.

Sound Power. Chant silently or aloud:

Hei Heng Hong Ah Xi Yi Weng You (pronounced *hay hung hawng*
  ah shee yee wung yoe)
Hei Heng Hong Ah Xi Yi Weng You
Hei Heng Hong Ah Xi Yi Weng You
Hei Heng Hong Ah Xi Yi Weng You
Hei Heng Hong Ah Xi Yi Weng You
Hei Heng Hong Ah Xi Yi Weng You...

Mind Power. As you chant, visualize a beam of golden light starting from the Hui Yin acupuncture point in the perineum and flowing up through the seven Soul Houses to the Bai Hui acupuncture point at the top of the head. From there it flows down in front of the spinal column through the Wai Jiao and back to the Hui Yin acupuncture point.

Stop reading now. Chant and visualize for ten minutes.

This energy circle is extremely powerful. The longer you chant and the more often you chant, the better. There is no time limit. You can chant this mantra silently all day long. The benefits for your healing cannot be expressed enough.

When I received this *Divine Soul Song of Yin Yang Energy Circle for Healing*, I was deeply moved and touched. I understood from the bottom of my heart that the Divine had released one of the most important healing treasures and tools to empower humanity to self-heal. I told the Divine, "Thank you so much for this sacred teaching and practice. I am extremely honored to receive it. I am extremely privileged to be able to release it to humanity."

The Divine continued:

There is another sacred wisdom and practice I am going to teach you now. This is the sacred and secret matter circle for rejuvenation and long life. The Divine Soul Song for this circle is:

> *You Weng Yi Xi Ah Hong Heng Hei* (pronounced *yoe wung yee shee ah hawng hung hay*)
> *You Weng Yi Xi Ah Hong Heng Hei*
> *You Weng Yi Xi Ah Hong Heng Hei*
> *You Weng Yi Xi Ah Hong Heng Hei . . .*

When you sing this Soul Song or chant these words, the circle starts from the genital area, goes in front of and then inside the tailbone, then up through the spinal cord to the brain and the Bai Hui acupuncture point in the crown chakra.[6] *Then it goes down through the brain to the roof of the mouth, then down the middle of the body through the other Soul Houses to the first Soul House just above the Hui Yin acupuncture point and perineum. This is the most important matter circle in the body.* (See figure 11.)

This matter circle is one of the most powerful treasures and tools that the Divine has given to humanity to empower us to rejuvenate and prolong life. Ancient Tao practice has shared some of the most sacred practices and phrases for rejuvenation and longevity. They are:

Shen Sheng Jing. "Shen" means *kidneys*. "Sheng" means *produce*. "Jing" means *matter*. "Shen Sheng Jing" (pronounced *shun shung jing*) means *kidneys create matter*.

---

[6] The Bai Hui acupuncture point, pronounced *bye hway*, is in the center of the top of the head. All the yang energy in the body gathers at the Bai Hui acupuncture point.

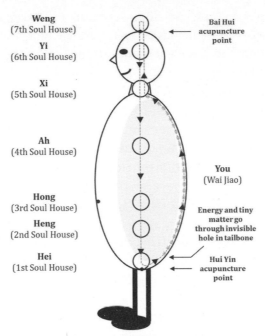

You Weng Yi Xi Ah Hong Heng Hei
(pronounced *yoe wung yee shee ah hawng hung hay*)

FIGURE 11. Most important matter circle in the body

Jing Sheng Sui. "Sui" means *spinal cord*. "Jing Sheng Sui" (pronounced *jing shung sway*) means *matter creates spinal cord*. This is to share with the spiritual seeker that jing moves into the spinal cord through an invisible hole in front of the spinal column.

Sui Chong Nao. "Chong" means *fulfill*. "Nao" means *brain*. "Sui Chong Nao" (pronounced *sway chawng now*) means the *spinal cord fills the brain*. This means the matter and energy of the spinal cord nourish and support the brain.

Nao Shen Ming. "Shen Ming" means *enlightenment*. "Nao Shen Ming" (pronounced *now shun ming*) means *mind reaches enlightenment*.

Lian Jing Hua Qi. "Lian" means *cook*. "Jing" means *matter*. "Hua" means *transform*. "Qi" means *energy*. "Lian Jing Hua Qi" (pronounced *lyen jing hwah chee*) means *transform matter to energy*. This means to transform jing to qi.

The matter produced from the kidneys moves to the tailbone and goes into the spinal cord. This is the process of Lian Jing Hua Qi.

Lian Qi Hua Shen. "Shen" here represents *the soul.* "Lian Qi Hua Shen" (pronounced *lyen chee hwah shun*) means *transform energy to the essence of soul.* This process is to move the energy from the spinal cord to the brain and to transform the soul.

Lian Shen Huan Xu. "Xu" means *emptiness and purity.* "Lian Shen Huan Xu" (pronounced *lyen shun hwahn shü)* means *transform the soul to purity.* This process happens from the head to the heart.

Lian Xu Huan Tao. "Tao" is *the Source.* Where is Tao inside the body? The Zhong is Tao inside the body. The Zhong is located in the back half of the lower abdomen and includes four sacred points and areas: Hui Yin acupuncture point, Kun Gong area, Ming Men acupuncture point, and Wei Lü tailbone area. (See figure 12.) "Lian Xu Huan Tao" (pronounced *lyen shü hwahn dow*) means *transform purity to absolute purity*

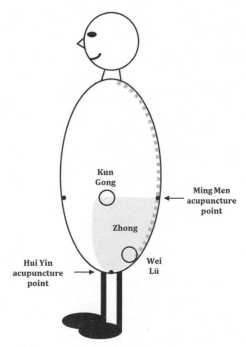

FIGURE 12. Zhong and four sacred areas

in order to reach Tao. This is the process of moving energy from the heart through the center of the body via the Soul Houses to the Zhong.

The above sacred phrases have exactly shared the sacred matter circle that the Divine gave to me. We chant:

> *You Weng Yi Xi Ah Hong Heng Hei* (pronounced *yoe wung yee shee ah hawng hung hay*)
> *You Weng Yi Xi Ah Hong Heng Hei*
> *You Weng Yi Xi Ah Hong Heng Hei*
> *You Weng Yi Xi Ah Hong Heng Hei*
> *You Weng Yi Xi Ah Hong Heng Hei*
> *You Weng Yi Xi Ah Hong Heng Hei*
> *You Weng Yi Xi Ah Hong Heng Hei...*

When you chant, visualize a golden beam forming a circle. The circle of the golden beam rotates from the Hui Yin acupuncture point to the tailbone through the center of the spinal cord to the top of the head to the Bai Hui acupuncture point. Then it flows down the center of the body through the seven Soul Houses back to the Hui Yin area.

Stop reading now. Chant and meditate for ten minutes.

> *You Weng Yi Xi Ah Hong Heng Hei* (pronounced *yoe wung yee shee ah hawng hung hay*)
> *You Weng Yi Xi Ah Hong Heng Hei*
> *You Weng Yi Xi Ah Hong Heng Hei*
> *You Weng Yi Xi Ah Hong Heng Hei*
> *You Weng Yi Xi Ah Hong Heng Hei*
> *You Weng Yi Xi Ah Hong Heng Hei*
> *You Weng Yi Xi Ah Hong Heng Hei...*

This is a very sacred practice. It summarizes much ancient sacred wisdom and practice. I would like to really emphasize this practice. There is no time limit. Chant as much as you can. Every time you chant you are rejuvenating. You are prolonging your life.

Words are not enough to express the benefits.

Thoughts are not enough to explain the profound power of this most important matter circle.

I have introduced the divine energy circle and divine matter circle of the *Divine Soul Song of Yin Yang*. This is only one of the Divine Soul Songs that I taught in the book, *Divine Soul Songs: Sacred Practical Treasures to Heal, Rejuvenate, and Transform You, Humanity, Mother Earth, and All Universes*.[7] I have received many more sacred Divine and Tao Soul Songs in the last eight years. You can use the *Divine Soul Songs* book to study and practice in order to transform all of your life.

Heal the Spiritual, Mental, Emotional, and Physical Bodies Together

I would like to share with every reader a sacred way to practice with the most important energy circle and the most important matter circle together.

Apply the Four Power Techniques:

Body Power. Sit up straight. Gently touch the tip of your tongue to the roof of your mouth. Place one palm over your navel. Place the other palm over the Ming Men acupuncture point.

Soul Power. Say *hello* to inner souls:

> *Dear soul mind body of the most important energy circle and the*
>   *most important matter circle,*
> *I love you both, honor you both, and appreciate you both.*
> *You have the power to heal and rejuvenate my spiritual, mental,*
>   *emotional, and physical bodies.*
> *You have the power to boost energy, stamina, vitality, and immunity,*
>   *and to prolong life.*
> *Do a good job!*
> *Thank you.*

---

[7] Toronto/New York: Heaven's Library/Atria Books, 2009.

Say *hello* to outer souls:

> *Dear Divine,*
> *Dear Tao, The Source,*
> *Dear countless planets, stars, galaxies, and universes,*
> *Dear all healing angels, archangels, ascended masters, gurus,*
>   *lamas, kahunas, holy saints, Taoist saints, other saints, buddhas,*
>   *bodhisattvas, and all kinds of spiritual fathers and mothers,*
> *Please forgive my ancestors and me for all of the mistakes we have*
>   *made in all lifetimes.*
> *Please remove soul mind body blockages from my spiritual, mental,*
>   *emotional, and physical bodies.*
> *In order to be forgiven I will serve unconditionally.*
> *To chant, meditate, and offer all kinds of acts of kindness, including*
>   *offering love, forgiveness, compassion, light, generosity, sincerity,*
>   *honesty, and more, are important services to offer humanity.*
> *I will offer these services a lot.*
> *Thank you. Thank you. Thank you.*

Sound Power. The sacred practice is to chant the divine energy circle four times and then to chant the divine matter circle four times.

> *Hei Heng Hong Ah Xi Yi Weng You* (pronounced *hay hung hawng*
>   *ah shee yee wung yoe*)
> *Hei Heng Hong Ah Xi Yi Weng You*
> *Hei Heng Hong Ah Xi Yi Weng You*
> *Hei Heng Hong Ah Xi Yi Weng You*
>
> *You Weng Yi Xi Ah Hong Heng Hei* (pronounced *yoe wung yee shee*
>   *ah hawng hung hay*)
> *You Weng Yi Xi Ah Hong Heng Hei*…
> *You Weng Yi Xi Ah Hong Heng Hei*
> *You Weng Yi Xi Ah Hong Heng Hei*

The message of practicing this sacred energy and matter circle four times each in alternation is:

Heal. Heal. Heal. Heal.
Younger. Younger. Younger. Younger.

or

Heal. Heal. Heal. Heal.
Rejuvenate. Rejuvenate. Rejuvenate. Rejuvenate.

or

Heal. Heal. Heal. Heal.
Longevity. Longevity. Longevity. Longevity.

This sacred practice of the energy and matter circles together is the priceless treasure that the Divine gave humanity to empower us for healing, rejuvenation, prolonging life, and transforming all life.

Since I have received this divine sacred teaching and practice, my teachers and I have shared it with hundreds of thousands of people worldwide. People truly enjoy chanting these sacred circles and experiencing their power. Many soul healing miracles have been produced through this sacred chanting.

Practice. Practice. Practice.
Receive more and more benefits.
Heal yourself.
Heal your loved ones.
Heal humanity.
Heal all souls.
Rejuvenate.
Prolong life.
Move in the direction of immortality.

Hao!

Divine and Tao Healing

IN JULY 2003 the Divine chose me as a servant of humanity and the servant, vehicle, and channel of the Divine. I was given the honor and authority to offer divine healing and blessing services. Since then I have offered divine services, including Divine Karma Cleansing, Soul Mind Body Transplants, and more, to hundreds of thousands of people worldwide. Now I have created more than thirty divine servants, vehicles, and channels worldwide who are my Worldwide Representatives and Divine Channels. They also offer divine healing and blessing services. We are training nearly four hundred students worldwide to become divine servants, vehicles, and channels.

We have also created more than four thousand Divine Healing Hands Soul Healers and hundreds of divine soul communicators worldwide. In this chapter I will introduce some of the most important divine services. There are many more divine services in addition to those I will introduce here.

Divine and Tao Soul Mind Body Healing and Transmission System

I started to offer divine treasures to humanity in 2003. In 2008 I was given the honor and authority from Tao to offer Tao frequency treasures to humanity.

What is the Divine and Tao Soul Mind Body Healing and Transmission System? It is a breakthrough soul healing system for humanity. In my

Soul Power Series book, *Divine Soul Mind Body Healing and Transmission System: The Divine Way to Heal You, Humanity, Mother Earth, and All Universes,*[8] I explained this extraordinary healing system and its benefits.

In this book I will give a brief explanation of this system.

In my more than twenty years of teaching soul wisdom, knowledge, and practical soul techniques, I have taught that everyone and everything is made of soul, mind, and body. In ancient times there was a renowned spiritual statement:

Wan wu jie you ling

"Wan" means *ten thousand*. In Chinese, "ten thousand" represents *all* or *every*. "Wu" means *thing*. "Jie" means *all*. "You" means *has*. "Ling" means *soul*. Therefore, *Wan wu jie you ling* (pronounced *wahn woo jyeh yoe ling*) means *everything has a soul*.

Living things have a soul. For example, human beings, animals, insects, bacteria, viruses, trees, and flowers have souls. *Wan wu jie you ling* emphasizes that *inanimate things also have souls*.

For example, a mountain, a river, a tree, a house, a street, the name of a business, a relationship, planets, stars, galaxies, universes, and this book, all have souls.

A human being is made of soul, mind, and body. An animal is made of soul, mind, and body. A tree is made of soul, mind, and body. An ocean, mountain, Mother Earth, and every planet, star, galaxy, and universe is made of soul, mind, and body.

Soul is spirit. Mind is consciousness. Body includes energy and matter.

What is the Divine and Tao Soul Mind Body Healing and Transmission System? This divine soul healing system includes Soul Mind Body Transplants. Soul Transplant means the Divine or Tao creates a new light being. This light being is a new divine or Tao soul that replaces an original soul of one of your organs or bodily systems or parts of the body or energy centers or Soul Houses or spaces such as the Wai Jiao or more, or a "cell package" of new divine or Tao souls that replace the original souls of the cells, cell units, DNA, RNA, tiny matter, and spaces

---

[8] Toronto/New York: Heaven's Library/Atria Books, 2009.

between the cells of one of your organs or bodily systems or parts of the body or energy centers or Soul Houses or spaces such as the Wai Jiao or more, in order to heal and transform the soul or souls. *Heal and transform the soul first; then healing and transformation of the mind and body and every aspect of life will follow.*

The Divine and Tao Soul Mind Body Healing and Transmission System is often given for a health condition. Then the appropriate Soul Transplant or Transplants will be given by the Divine or Tao as needed for the health condition.

I will explain Mind Transplants and Body Transplants later in this chapter.

Before offering Soul Mind Body Transplants for the requested organ, system, part of the body, or health condition, the Divine or Tao offers sickness karma cleansing. Sickness karma is the negative karma that a person carries from all lifetimes, which is the root cause of the current sickness. In sickness karma cleansing, the Divine and Tao remove the karma associated with the sickness. The person's mistakes related to the sickness are forgiven by the Divine and Tao. This is a tremendous blessing.

I will not discuss negative karma in detail in this book. In some of the major books in my Soul Power Series, I have explained negative karma and Divine and Tao Karma Cleansing in great detail. I sincerely recommend that you read them. It is very important to understand negative karma and how it affects your physical life and your soul journey. It is most important to learn how to self-clear negative karma in order to transform every aspect of your life.

One of my authority books is *The Power of Soul: The Way to Heal, Rejuvenate, Transform, and Enlighten All Life.*[9] The longest chapter in this book is entirely about karma.

Karma is the record of services. Karma is the term used in Buddhist teaching. Taoists use the term *de* (pronounced *duh*). Christians use the term "deed." Many other spiritual beings use the term "virtue." Karma, *de*, deed, and virtue are different words for the same thing. To understand karma is to understand all of these words.

---

[9] Toronto/New York: Heaven's Library/Atria Books, 2009.

Karma can be divided into good karma and bad karma. Good karma is the record of one's good services in this life and in all past lives. Good services include love, care, compassion, sincerity, honesty, generosity, kindness, purity, and all other kinds of good service. Bad karma is a record of one's unpleasant services, such as killing, harming, taking advantage of others, cheating, stealing, and all other kinds of unpleasant service.

The power and significance of karma can be summarized in one sentence:

**Karma is the root cause of success and failure
in every aspect of life.**

You could also receive great benefits from reading my book *Divine Soul Mind Body Healing and Transmission System: The Divine Way to Heal You, Humanity, Mother Earth, and All Universes.*[10] In this book I have explained all kinds of soul mind body blockages in detail. I have explained many times that soul blockages are all kinds of negative karma. Mind blockages include negative mind-sets, negative beliefs, negative attitudes, ego, attachments, and more. Body blockages are energy blockages and matter blockages.

In *Divine Soul Mind Body Healing and Transmission System* I offer readers forty-six permanent divine treasures to help them self-clear their soul mind body blockages. These are priceless treasures that you can receive simply by reading the book, and then use to create your own soul healing miracles.

Another major book in my Soul Power Series is *Divine Transformation: The Divine Way to Self-clear Karma to Transform Your Health, Relationships, Finances, and More.*[11] In this book I give every reader further practical soul healing techniques and thirty more permanent divine treasures to self-clear karma in order to transform every aspect of life.

The books of my Soul Power Series have helped humanity create thousands of heart-touching and moving stories. I encourage you to

---

[10] Toronto/New York: Heaven's Library/Atria Books, 2009.

[11] Toronto/New York: Heaven's Library/Atria Books, 2010.

read, practice with, and receive the permanent divine and Tao treasures from these books to transform all of your life.

Returning now to Soul Mind Body Transplants, Mind Transplant means the Divine or Tao creates another light being that carries Divine or Tao consciousness. This light being replaces an original consciousness of your systems, organs, cells, cell units, DNA, RNA, tiny matter, spaces, or more, in order to heal and transform the mind of the systems, organs, cells, cell units, DNA, RNA, tiny matter, spaces, or more by helping to remove negative mind-sets, negative attitudes, negative beliefs, ego, attachments, and other mind blockages.

Body Transplant means the Divine or Tao creates another light being that carries Divine or Tao energy and tiny matter. This light being replaces the original energy and tiny matter of your systems, organs, cells, cell units, DNA, RNA, tiny matter, spaces, or more, in order to heal and transform the energy and tiny matter.

For example, Divine Soul Mind Body Transplants of Heart include three light beings: Divine Heart Soul Transplant, Divine Heart Mind Transplant, and Divine Heart Body Transplant. These three light beings join as one when they are transmitted to the recipient.

Since July 2003 I have offered hundreds of thousands of Divine and Tao Soul Mind Body Transplants of systems, organs, parts of the body, and more. These Divine and Tao treasures have created thousands and hundreds of thousands of soul healing miracles.

I welcome you to visit my YouTube channel, www.YouTube.com/ zhigangsha, to view hundreds of soul healing miracle videos.

Here is an inspiring story from a psychologist who received a Divine Soul Mind Body Healing and Transmission System for cancer. She practiced dedicatedly and was blessed with tremendous results.

Stage four lymphoma cleared in soul healing miracle

I am a teacher, healer, and consultant with a doctorate in applied psychology. In 2009 I was diagnosed with stage four lymphoma while also in a serious clinical depression and with very limited financial resources. It was quite an overwhelming situation for me. During that time I was very blessed to be introduced to the teachings of Dr. and Master Zhi Gang Sha. I learned to sing the Divine Soul Songs that were being brought through Master Sha and began to practice. Singing these songs uplifted me enough to begin to deal with my situation.

Within a few short weeks, my depression lifted. Very soon after that, I received a Divine Soul Mind Body Healing and Transmission System from Master Sha, which included Divine Karma Cleansing for the cancer and Soul Mind Body Transplants for healing. I chanted very dedicatedly to activate my divine treasures, as required by this divine healing system. My doctor administered a non-chemo drug therapy during this time to help alleviate pain and "keep the cancer at bay." He indicated that without chemo, I would need this treatment every six months.

I'm happy to say that with regular practice, three-and-a-half months after receiving the divine soul healing, test results demonstrated the cancer had cleared. Furthermore, I have needed no medical treatment for cancer since then, for over three years now, to my doctor's delight and surprise! I continue to chant and practice soul healing, Soul Power, and Soul Mind Body Medicine techniques as much as possible and I have become a Divine Soul Healer through the training and transmissions offered by Master Sha. As I grow in wisdom, more is revealed. As I grow in mastery, healing and transformation happen on the spot—instantly. I now experience soul healing miracles regularly, and I'm confident that you can also!

In summary, the teachings, practices, and blessings delivered by Master Sha have helped to transform my life in every way. For this and more, I am extremely and deeply grateful.

Marsha Valutis
Florida

Now I am going to offer four major treasures to every reader as a gift from Heaven. They are named:

**Tao Love Golden Light Ball and Golden Liquid Spring
Soul Mind Body Transplants**

**Tao Forgiveness Golden Light Ball and Golden Liquid Spring
Soul Mind Body Transplants**

**Tao Compassion Golden Light Ball and Golden Liquid Spring
Soul Mind Body Transplants**

**Tao Light Golden Light Ball and Golden Liquid Spring
Soul Mind Body Transplants**

My books are totally unique. The Divine and Tao download their priceless permanent soul treasures to readers as they read these books. In the ten books of my Soul Power Series, the Divine and Tao have pre-programmed Divine and Tao Soul Mind Body Transplants as treasured gifts and have offered them to humanity. I will continue to offer this divine service in every book of my Soul Healing Miracles Series.

Simply relax and continue to read the book. When you read the appropriate paragraphs and pause for a minute, the above Tao gifts (and others later in this book) will be transmitted to your soul. When I ask you to stop to receive the treasures, you will then receive the treasures. They come into your crown chakra, which is located at the top of your head, and move through your Soul Houses to reside in your lower abdomen. For additional information about receiving Divine and Tao soul treasures, please read the earlier section, "How to Receive the Divine and Tao Soul Downloads Offered in the Books of the Soul Healing Miracles Series."

After receiving the four permanent Tao treasures, you can invoke any or all of them to offer healing and blessing to any part of the body. You also can invoke these treasures to radiate to offer healing and blessing to others. To do so, simply "say *hello*" to invoke these treasures:

Dear all my divine and Tao treasures,
I love you, honor you, and appreciate you.
Please turn on to offer a soul healing blessing as appropriate to
    _____ (name the person) *for* _____ (state your
    request).
I am very grateful.
Thank you.

Then chant:

Divine treasures heal and rejuvenate _____ (name the person
Thank you.

for several minutes. The longer and the more often you practice, the
better the results the person could receive.

Soul healing is not limited by time or space. You can apply your
permanent divine and Tao treasures to offer soul healing blessings in
person or remotely.

Now I am offering the first set of priceless permanent Tao soul treasures to you.

Prepare! Sit up straight. Close your eyes. Totally relax. Put both palms
on your lower abdomen.

Tao Love Golden Light Ball and Golden Liquid Spring
Soul Mind Body Transplants

Transmission!

Congratulations! You are extremely blessed.

The Tao Love Soul Transplant is the soul of Tao love.
The Tao Love Mind Transplant is the consciousness of Tao love.

The Tao Love Body Transplant is the energy and tiny matter of Tao love.

I cannot emphasize enough that *love melts all blockages and transforms all life.* Let us apply these treasures right away to receive their healing and blessing. I will lead you to apply the Tao Love Soul Mind Body Transplants to heal the spiritual body.

Heal the Spiritual Body

Apply the Four Power Techniques:

Body Power. Sit up straight. Place the tip of your tongue gently on the roof of your mouth. Place one palm below your navel on your lower abdomen. Place the other palm over your heart.

Soul Power. Say *hello* to inner souls:

> *Dear soul mind body of my spiritual body,*
> *I love you, honor you, and appreciate you.*
> *You have the power to heal yourself.*
> *Do a great job!*
> *Dear Tao Love Golden Light Ball and Golden Liquid Spring Soul*
>   *Mind Body Transplants,*
> *I love you, honor you, and appreciate you.*
> *Please heal my spiritual body.*
> *Thank you both.*

Say *hello* to outer souls:

> *Dear Divine,*
> *Dear Tao, The Source,*
> *Dear countless planets, stars, galaxies, and universes,*
> *Dear all healing angels, archangels, ascended masters, gurus,*
>   *lamas, kahunas, holy saints, Taoist saints, other saints, buddhas,*
>   *bodhisattvas, and all kinds of spiritual fathers and mothers,*

> *Please forgive my ancestors and me for all of the mistakes that we*
> *have made in all lifetimes.*
> *Please remove soul mind body blockages from my spiritual body.*
> *In order to be forgiven I will serve unconditionally.*
> *To chant, meditate, and offer all kinds of acts of kindness, including*
> *love, forgiveness, compassion, light, generosity, sincerity, honesty,*
> *and more, are important services to offer humanity.*
> *I will offer these services a lot.*
> *Thank you. Thank you. Thank you.*

Mind Power. Visualize golden light radiating in the heart area as you chant.

Sound Power. Chant silently or aloud:

> *Tao Love Soul Mind Body Transplants heal and bless my spiritual*
> *body. Thank you.*
> *Tao Love Soul Mind Body Transplants heal and bless my spiritual*
> *body. Thank you.*
> *Tao Love Soul Mind Body Transplants heal and bless my spiritual*
> *body. Thank you.*
> *Tao Love Soul Mind Body Transplants heal and bless my spiritual*
> *body. Thank you…*

Stop reading. Practice and chant for ten minutes. For chronic or life-threatening conditions chant two hours or more per day. You can add all of your chanting time together to total at least two hours. In fact, there is no time limit. You can chant anytime, anywhere. The more you chant, the better the results you could receive.

You can apply Tao Love Golden Light Ball and Golden Liquid Spring Soul Mind Body Transplants to offer healing to your mental body, emotional body, and physical body. Use the Four Power Techniques in a similar way to do the soul self-healing.

There is a spiritual reason for every significant blockage in our lives. This includes blockages in health, emotions, relationships, finances, business, and more. Soul healing can be applied in every aspect of life because everyone and everything has a soul. Enjoy these stories about applying soul healing blessings, teachings, and practices to transform financial blockages.

Financial blessings can come to your life too!

As soon as the opportunity to watch the Soul Healing on Demand video for financial blessing arose, I immediately signed up for it. My finances are usually quite tight, and my deepest wish is to receive more Divine Karma Cleansing and other divine services this year.

At first I was able to watch the video only a few times due to a slow Internet connection. The video would take a very long time to load.

My aunt contacted me to tell me that some people owed her money, and she told them that they should pay the money back to my bank account! In three months it has totaled 950 euros. That is a huge amount of money for me, and has enabled me to register for more Divine and Tao services.

Then my Internet connection was changed and I was able to watch the video more often. Just today (exactly one month after the last payment from my aunt), I came back to work after my holidays. I received my paycheck, and it was almost double the usual amount! Due to a change in the accounting system, everyone received more pay and will receive more money every month. This change started from January, so I received about 900 Euros more.

I am so extremely grateful and can only encourage everyone to sign up for this service and watch the video daily and practice as often as you can. It really, really works! Financial blessings can come to your life too!

Nina K.
Germany

Soul Power techniques hasten property sale

I'm a real estate agent in Hawaii, and in early January 2013 I received a listing to sell a condo property. I received several inquiries and appointments for the property from potential buyers. However, I received no offers there-after. By the fourth month I still had no offers, which didn't seem right in a strong sellers' market. I went to the property and brought my CD player to play the Divine Soul Song Love, Peace and Harmony *and also placed my Divine Healing Hands book in the doorway entrance. I did an invocation and chanted my Soul Language and asked the Divine Healing Hands treasures in the book to stay turned on until the right buyers were found.*

Later that same day I received our first cash offer! Then I received another offer, and then another one—all within a few days, followed by other serious inquiries. The first two offers were very strong cash buyers, which enabled the negotiation process and ultimately resulted in an additional $45,000 above the original asking price. The escrow transaction was very smooth and we closed the deal in three weeks!

Thank you so much, Master Sha, for empowering us with your practices. Your teaching and wisdom have completely transformed my entire life, and my loved ones receive the healing blessings and benefits as well. I thank you, I love you, and I honor you from the bottom of my heart forever and all eternity. I am so elated with joy and happiness to have met you again to serve in this lifetime.

Orlena
Honolulu, Hawaii, U.S.A.

Heal the Mental Body

Now I will offer the second set of priceless permanent treasures as a gift to every reader.

Prepare! Sit up straight. Close your eyes. Totally relax. Put both palms on your lower abdomen.

**Tao Forgiveness Golden Light Ball and Golden Liquid Spring
Soul Mind Body Transplants**

Transmission!

Congratulations! You are extremely blessed.

The Tao Forgiveness Soul Transplant is the soul of Tao forgiveness.

The Tao Forgiveness Mind Transplant is the consciousness of Tao forgiveness.

The Tao Forgiveness Body Transplant is the energy and tiny matter of Tao forgiveness.

Forgiveness is the key for self-clearing negative karma. Negative karma is the root blockage in every aspect of life, including health, emotions, relationships, finances, business, and more.

These Tao Forgiveness treasures are priceless. They could create soul healing miracles beyond comprehension. They will be with your soul forever. Value and honor the treasures from the bottom of your heart.

I will lead you to apply the Four Power Techniques and Tao Forgiveness Golden Light Ball and Golden Liquid Spring Soul Mind Body Transplants to heal the mental body. Forgiveness brings inner joy and inner peace to all life. I emphasize again that love and forgiveness are the golden keys to transform all life.

Body Power. Sit up straight. Place the tip of your tongue gently on the roof of your mouth. Place one palm below your navel. Place the other palm on the crown chakra at the top of your head.

Soul Power. Say *hello* to inner souls:

> *Dear soul mind body of my mental body,*
> *I love you, honor you, and appreciate you.*
> *You have the power to heal yourself.*
> *Do a great job!*
> *Thank you.*
> *Dear Tao Forgiveness Golden Light Ball and Golden Liquid Spring*
>   *Soul Mind Body Transplants,*
> *I love you, honor you, and appreciate you.*
> *Please heal my mental body.*
> *Thank you.*

Say *hello* to outer souls:

> *Dear Divine,*
> *Dear Tao, The Source,*
> *Dear countless planets, stars, galaxies, and universes,*
> *Dear all healing angels, archangels, ascended masters, gurus,*
>   *lamas, kahunas, holy saints, Taoist saints, other saints, buddhas,*
>   *bodhisattvas, and all kinds of spiritual fathers and mothers,*
> *Please forgive my ancestors and me for all of the mistakes that we*
>   *have made in all lifetimes.*
> *Please remove soul mind body blockages from my mental body.*
> *In order to be forgiven I will serve unconditionally.*
> *To chant, meditate, and offer all kinds of acts of kindness, including*
>   *offering love, forgiveness, compassion, light, generosity, sincerity,*
>   *honesty, and more, are important services to offer humanity.*
> *I will offer these services a lot.*
> *Thank you. Thank you. Thank you.*

Mind Power. Visualize golden light radiating in your head as you chant.

Sound Power. Chant silently or aloud:

> *Tao Forgiveness Soul Mind Body Transplants heal and bless my*
>   *mental body. Thank you.*
> *Tao Forgiveness Soul Mind Body Transplants heal and bless my*
>   *mental body. Thank you.*
> *Tao Forgiveness Soul Mind Body Transplants heal and bless my*
>   *mental body. Thank you.*
> *Tao Forgiveness Soul Mind Body Transplants heal and bless my*
>   *mental body. Thank you...*

Stop reading. Practice and chant for ten minutes. For chronic or life-threatening conditions, chant two hours or more per day. You can add all of your chanting time together to total at least two hours per day. In fact, there is no time limit. You can chant anytime, anywhere. The more you chant, the better the results you could receive.

You can apply Tao Forgiveness Golden Light Ball and Golden Liquid Spring Soul Mind Body Transplants to offer healing to your spiritual body, emotional body, and physical body. Use the Four Power Techniques in a similar way to do the soul self-healing.

Soul healing miracle for obsessive-compulsive disorder

On June 8, 2004, I met Dr. and Master Zhi Gang Sha. My life was deeply transformed forever because on this day the true healing of my obsessive-compulsive disorder (OCD) began. On this day, I knew I would be healed.

Before this day, I had suffered greatly for over half my life in my health, relationships, finances, business, spiritual journey, and more. At the age of ten, I developed negative, obsessive thoughts, fears, worry, and anxiety that drove me to compulsions of counting and touching things four times or in multiples of four. After being diagnosed with OCD, I started taking medication. I forced behavioral changes so as not to perform the counting or thinking obsessions through willpower and self-therapy as I had not heard of cognitive behavior therapy at that time. Many other obsessions and compulsions continued, such as not being able to let things go, always wanting to face fear, ego, pride, and a rigid mind that created a lot of suffering in every aspect of my life. I suffered from the side effects of the medication I took, which included being constantly tired and having dry mouth. I suffered because I was supposed to be on medication every day for the rest of my life as conventional medicine has no cure for OCD. I suffered because I could not live or even achieve my dreams.

At this sacred Soul Retreat in June 2004, I received Divine Personal Karma Cleansing, many Divine Soul Downloads, and a Divine Order for Soul Enlightenment. I learned soul secrets, wisdom, knowledge, and practices for soul self-healing and the soul journey. I learned that I had the power to heal myself and, more importantly, I was given the divine tools to do so. I left this retreat feeling like I had driven through a divine car wash and come out cleaner than ever before.

Afterward I practiced Master Sha's Divine Soul Healing System a lot. I joined the free teleclasses and tuition-based trainings. I attended more events. I received more divine blessings. When Master Sha received the authority and offered Divine Soul Operation for the first time in January 2005, I knew I was healed. I worked with my conventional medical doctor to get off of my medication over the months that followed. On June 8, 2005 I totally stopped my OCD medication!

In February 2009 I was approved for normal health insurance coverage as given to a healthy person. Due to my history, I was previously paying $6000 per year in health insurance premiums just to have coverage. This was a very special moment in my life. It was also an incredible financial blessing.

On this journey with Master Sha, I have experienced the most amazing joy, love, forgiveness, compassion, light, gratitude, and inner freedom. I have rediscovered the Divine, Tao, and The Source in ways that are beyond a dream. Most important, I have found my teacher, master, and spiritual father, Master Sha. I have been given the honor, privilege, and authority to be a Disciple and Worldwide Representative of Master Sha, which I believe is the greatest honor anyone could ever receive.

There are no words to express what I feel in my heart. I wish for all to receive what I have received. I wish for all to achieve their dreams. I wish for all to receive the soul healing miracles they need in order to become the best unconditional universal servants they can be.

With love and blessings,

Master David Lusch
Germany

Never give up!

I suffered from a serious and chronic mental disorder. It was not so easy, because I couldn't see or feel in advance when it would strike again. I stayed several times in hospitals for people with this illness. The doors are kept locked and everyone receives very strong medication.

In my case, I would always be discharged from the hospital after a few weeks and then try to go on with my daily life on my own, until the next episode.

In 2012 Master Sha visited a city in my area. It was great. I applied to become a Divine Healing Hands Soul Healer and took part in the certification training. In 2013 I was very, very happy to register for the Source Soul Mind Body Science Healing and Transmission System and received Karma Cleansing for my condition.

Since then I feel free and I am full of gratitude.

And I want to share: Never give up!

Mrs. B.
Germany

Heal the Emotional Body

Now I am delighted to offer the third set of extraordinary treasures to every reader.

Compassion boosts energy, stamina, vitality, and immunity. Compassion has incredible power to transform all life.

Prepare! Sit up straight. Close your eyes. Totally relax. Put both palms on your lower abdomen.

Tao Compassion Golden Light Ball and Golden Liquid Spring Soul Mind Body Transplants

Transmission!

Congratulations! You are extremely blessed.

The Tao Compassion Soul Transplant is the soul of Tao compassion.

The Tao compassion Mind Transplant is the consciousness of Tao compassion.

The Tao Compassion Body Transplant is the energy and tiny matter of Tao compassion.

Now I will lead you to apply the Four Power Techniques and Tao Compassion Golden Light Ball and Golden Liquid Spring Soul Mind Body Transplants for healing the emotional body. Imbalances in the emotional body include anger, depression, anxiety, worry, grief, sadness, fear, guilt, unworthiness, shame, lack of self-love, and more.

Body Power. Sit up straight. Place the tip of your tongue gently against the roof of your mouth. Place one palm below the navel. Place the other palm on the Message Center[12] in the center of your chest.

Soul Power. Say *hello* to inner souls:

> *Dear soul mind body of my emotional body,*
> *I love you, honor you, and appreciate you.*
> *You have the power to heal yourself.*
> *Do a great job!*
> *Thank you.*
> *Dear Tao Compassion Golden Light Ball and Golden Liquid Spring*
>   *Soul Mind Body Transplants,*
> *I love you, honor you, and appreciate you.*
> *Please heal my emotional body.*
> *I am very grateful.*
> *Thank you.*

Say *hello* to outer souls:

> *Dear Divine,*
> *Dear Tao, The Source,*
> *Dear countless planets, stars, galaxies, and universes,*
> *Dear all healing angels, archangels, ascended masters, gurus,*
>   *lamas, kahunas, holy saints, Taoist saints, other saints, buddhas,*
>   *bodhisattvas, and all kinds of spiritual fathers and mothers,*
> *Please forgive my ancestors and me for all of the mistakes that we*
>   *have made in all lifetimes.*
> *Please remove soul mind body blockages from my emotional body.*

---

[12] The Message Center is a fist-sized energy center located in the center of the chest, behind the sternum. It is also known as the heart chakra. It is the key center for opening and developing spiritual channels. It is the love, forgiveness, compassion, and light center, the emotion center, the healing center, the life transformation center, the enlightenment center, and more.

In order to be forgiven I will serve unconditionally.
To chant, meditate, and offer all kinds of acts of kindness, including
*   love, forgiveness, compassion, light, generosity, sincerity, honesty,*
*   and more, are important services to offer humanity.*
I will offer these services a lot.
Thank you. Thank you. Thank you.

Mind Power. Visualize golden light radiating in and around your
Message Center as you chant.

Sound Power. Chant silently or aloud:

Tao Compassion Soul Mind Body Transplants heal and bless my
*   emotional body. Thank you.*
Tao Compassion Soul Mind Body Transplants heal and bless my
*   emotional body. Thank you.*
Tao Compassion Soul Mind Body Transplants heal and bless my
*   emotional body. Thank you.*
Tao Compassion Soul Mind Body Transplants heal and bless my
*   emotional body. Thank you . . .*

Stop reading. Please remember: do not skip the practices. They are to
ensure your healing, rejuvenation, and life transformation. Practice is
the key to create soul healing miracles.

Practice and chant for ten minutes. For chronic or life-threatening
conditions, chant two hours or more per day. You can add all of your
chanting time together to total at least two hours per day. In fact, there
is no time limit. You can chant anytime, anywhere. The more often you
chant and the longer you chant, the better the results you could receive.

You can apply Tao Compassion Golden Light Ball and Golden Liquid
Spring Soul Mind Body Transplants to offer healing to your spiritual
body, mental body, and physical body. Use the Four Power Techniques
in a similar way to do the soul self-healing.

Thousands of people worldwide have received heart-touching results from soul healing blessings and soul self-healing techniques. I am delighted to share these inspiring stories with you and every reader.

Addictions transformed by the power of soul healing

Dear Master Sha,

It has been almost four months since you gave me a healing blessing for my seven-year-old addictions. I cannot even begin to describe all of the amazing transformations that have happened in my life!

Since my healing and the amazing gift of the Divine Channel training, I have shifted so many things in my life. The craving for alcohol, cigarettes, and marijuana has popped up here and there in the last few weeks, but it is very different than it ever was before. It took several months before I even had a real "craving," and I've done as you told me to do when that happens—I turned on my treasures and chanted, and it has always made the craving go away within seconds!

The process of purification is a challenging one, but it is a path that I am happy to walk. I look forward to the process because I know that I will become a better person—a person that I can be proud of.

I am so grateful. Thank you, Master Sha.

Steve P.
Fort Collins, Colorado, U.S.A.

My depression vanished

In October 2008 I met Master Sha at a Soul Enlightenment Retreat. I had been suffering from depression my entire life and my life was not working out very well. I received personal and ancestral Divine Karma Cleansing from Master Sha at that retreat and within three days my life completely changed forever.

My depression vanished and my relationship with my parents was transformed. My friends noticed something different in me and, most important, I noticed the positive changes myself. I also felt the Soul Enlightenment Order given to us by Master Sha through the Divine. It was a powerful experience. I actually felt my soul moving up through my body!

I have been deeply blessed by the Divine and by Master Sha and I am extremely grateful. Thank you!

Andrea
Colorado, U.S.A.

Panic attacks healed by Divine Healing Hands blessings

Last October we were very busy in my office. A constant flow of patients came in for physicals, sick visits, and to receive their annual flu shots. The schedule for most providers was double booked all day, and left the medical assistants struggling to tend to the patients' needs and care.

One day, David, one of our medical assistants, left the office in the midst of his work, unable to handle the stress. He was overcome by a panic attack, shaken, and in tears. When I heard about the incident a few days later, I felt the need to help him. I approached David and asked if I could offer him a Divine Healing Hands soul healing blessing for his condition. He looked at me with a sign of hope in his eyes and a smile and said, "Yes, please." That night after work, he agreed to receive a healing blessing to help him better cope with his daily workflow.

The following Thursday, before going away to a Divine Healing Hands weekend retreat, I gave him another healing blessing and a CD of the Divine Soul Song Love, Peace and Harmony. *I asked him to play it 24/7 to assist him with his recovery.*

The next Monday, David told me that he was feeling much better. Listening to the CD was helping him sleep at night, calming his worries. After that conversation, we agreed to do one more healing session. He even confided in me that he had been considering leaving this busy practice because he was unable to deal with the stress and worried about having more panic attacks.

A few weeks later, another co-worker who had heard that David was doing much better, asked David if his doctor had prescribed any medicine to help him cope with his symptoms. David smiled and said, "No, I am fine now."

To this day, almost ten months later, David has not had any episodes of panic attacks. I am so happy that I was able to help a fellow co-worker.

Thank you, Divine. Thank you, Master Sha! We are so blessed.

Elise

Heal the Physical Body

Now I will offer the fourth set of permanent priceless treasures to every reader as a gift:

Tao Light Golden Light Ball and Golden Liquid Spring Soul Mind Body Transplants

Light heals, prevents all sickness, purifies and rejuvenates soul, heart, mind, and body, purifies and rejuvenates the spiritual, mental, emotional, and physical bodies, transforms relationships and finances, increases intelligence, opens spiritual channels, prolongs life, and brings success to all life.

Prepare! Sit up straight. Close your eyes. Totally relax. Put both palms on your lower abdomen.

Tao Light Golden Light Ball and Golden Liquid Spring Soul Mind Body Transplants

Transmission!

Congratulations! You are extremely blessed.

The Tao Light Soul Transplant is the soul of Tao light.

The Tao Light Mind Transplant is the consciousness of Tao light.

The Tao Light Body Transplant is the energy and tiny matter of Tao light.

Now I will lead you to apply the Four Power Techniques and Tao Light Golden Light Ball and Golden Liquid Spring Soul Mind Body Transplants for healing the physical body. The physical body includes all systems, all organs, all cells and cell units, all DNA and RNA, tiny matter inside the cells, and every part of the body.

Body Power. Sit up straight. Place the tip of your tongue gently to the roof of your mouth. Place one palm below the navel. Place the other palm on the Ming Men acupuncture point on your back, directly behind your navel. (See figure 8.)

Soul Power. Say *hello* to inner souls:

> *Dear soul mind body of my physical body,*
> *I love you, honor you, and appreciate you.*
> *You have the power to heal yourself.*
> *Do a great job!*
> *Thank you.*
> *Dear Tao Light Golden Light Ball and Golden Liquid Spring Soul*
>   *Mind Body Transplants,*
> *I love you, honor you, and appreciate you.*
> *Please heal my physical body.*

You may add specific requests for physical healing in this way:

> *Please heal my _____ (name your request).*
> *Thank you.*

Say *hello* to outer souls:

> *Dear Divine,*
> *Dear Tao, The Source,*
> *Dear countless planets, stars, galaxies, and universes,*
> *Dear all healing angels, archangels, ascended masters, gurus,*
>   *lamas, kahunas, holy saints, Taoist saints, other saints, buddhas,*
>   *bodhisattvas, and all kinds of spiritual fathers and mothers,*
> *Please forgive my ancestors and me for all of the mistakes that we*
>   *have made in all lifetimes.*
> *Please remove soul mind body blockages from my physical body.*
> *In order to be forgiven I will serve unconditionally.*
> *To chant, meditate, and offer all kinds of acts of kindness, including*
>   *love, forgiveness, compassion, light, generosity, sincerity, honesty,*
>   *and more, are important services to offer humanity.*
> *I will offer these services a lot.*
> *Thank you. Thank you. Thank you.*

Mind Power. Visualize golden light radiating in the area of your Ming Men acupuncture point as you chant.

Sound Power. Chant silently or aloud:

> *Tao Light priceless treasures heal and rejuvenate my physical body.*
>   *Thank you.*
> *Tao Light priceless treasures heal and rejuvenate my physical body.*
>   *Thank you.*
> *Tao Light priceless treasures heal and rejuvenate my physical body.*
>   *Thank you.*
> *Tao Light priceless treasures heal and rejuvenate my physical body.*
>   *Thank you…*

Stop reading. Practice and chant for ten minutes. For chronic or life-threatening conditions, chant two hours or more per day. You can add all of your chanting time together to total at least two hours per day. In fact, there is no time limit. You can chant anytime, anywhere. The more often you chant and the longer you chant, the better the results you could receive.

You can apply Tao Light Golden Light Ball and Golden Liquid Spring Soul Mind Body Transplants to offer healing to your spiritual body, mental body, and emotional body. Use the Four Power Techniques in a similar way to do the soul self-healing.

Tao Love, Forgiveness, Compassion, and Light Soul Mind Body Transplants are four heart-touching, moving, incredibly powerful, and extraordinary Source treasures to create soul healing miracles for the spiritual, mental, emotional, and physical bodies. Be sure to practice. If you have chronic or life-threatening conditions, practice a lot. It could take some time to transform your blockages. To receive soul treasures is a huge blessing. To gain the greatest benefit from them, you *must* practice.

Grateful to be cancer-free!

In May 2010 I was diagnosed with stage three breast cancer. The 10 cm tumor broke open during the needle biopsy. A week later I received a lumpectomy, but the surgeon was unable to get a good margin where it was attached to my chest wall. The radiology oncologist gave me a 5 to 15% chance they could get the cancer if I also did chemotherapy and six weeks of radiation treatment, but mentioned that the cancer most likely would return within five years. I decided instead to go to a clinic in Mexico for an alternative cancer treatment that friends of mine highly recommended.

I did well for a year but then started to feel extremely tired again. I had been under a lot of financial stress for a few years. My tumor marker, from blood test CA 15-3, which normally is less than 35, had shot up to 122! A 5 cm tumor was growing again in my breast and a total body bone scan in August 2012 showed bone cancer in four places.

After more tests, my oncologist said they wanted to do chemotherapy, a complete mastectomy, remove some of my chest wall, and then radiation, but there was nothing more they could do for the bone cancer except treat the extreme pain I would have! I turned down the chemo, surgery, and radiation. My doctors in Mexico increased my tonic, made some changes in my diet, and still felt we could get it under control. I was very ill.

In October 2012 a friend of my neighbors gave me a copy of Dr. and Master Sha's Divine Healing Hands *book and invited me to a healing evening at Master Sha's Soul Power Group in Kahului, Maui. Master Pam, one of Master Sha's Worldwide Representatives, was there from Honolulu and gave me a Crown Chakra Blessing that evening. I also started to do daily practices from the* Divine Transformation *book by Dr. Sha.*

Ten days after the Crown Chakra Blessing, I had a CT scan and the bone cancer was hardly detectable! On January 30, 2013 my CA 15-3 marker was 27.4 and doctors confirmed I'm cancer-free!

I am grateful beyond words for the blessings, teachings, and service. Thank You. Thank You. Thank You.

Marie Parker
Maui, Hawaii, U.S.A.

Injured cat's health restored with soul healing

We have been feeding this beautiful stray white cat for at least two years. He roams the neighborhood but spends most of his time at my parents' home. Periodically, he will wander off for a few weeks at a time. However, when he left at the beginning of the year, he was gone for two months. When he returned, he was very ill, had lost lots of hair and weight, and had been attacked. Everyone thought he would die very soon.

I felt a lot of compassion for him, so I gave him several Divine Healing Hands blessings. To everyone's surprise, he started to improve. Then he regressed a bit, so I repeated the blessings. His health is now completely restored without any medical care. He gained his weight back and he seems to be back to normal. Even though he's not my personal cat, I took the responsibility to feed him and keep an eye on him. For some reason, he has touched my heart. I am grateful for his healing because it was clear that he was suffering.

Tammy Simon
Thomasville, North Carolina, U.S.A.

Heal the Spiritual, Mental, Emotional, and Physical Bodies Together, from Head to Toe, Skin to Bone

Now let us apply these four sacred Tao Love, Tao Forgiveness, Tao Compassion, and Tao Light treasures to heal the spiritual, mental, emotional, and physical bodies together, from head to toe, skin to bone.

Apply the Four Power Techniques:

Body Power. Sit up straight. Place the tip of your tongue gently to the roof of your mouth. Place one palm below the navel. Place your other palm over the Ming Men acupuncture point on your back directly behind your navel. (See figure 8.)

Soul Power. Say *hello* to inner souls:

Dear soul mind body of my spiritual, mental, emotional, and
  physical bodies,
I love you, honor you, and appreciate you.
You have the power to heal yourselves.
Do a great job!
Thank you.
Dear Tao Love, Tao Forgiveness, Tao Compassion, and Tao Light
  Golden Light Ball and Golden Liquid Spring Soul Mind Body
  Transplants,
I love you, honor you, and appreciate you all.
Please heal my spiritual, mental, emotional, and physical bodies.
I am very grateful.
Thank you.

Say *hello* to outer souls:

Dear Divine,
Dear Tao, The Source,
Dear countless planets, stars, galaxies, and universes,
Dear all healing angels, archangels, ascended masters, gurus,
  lamas, kahunas, holy saints, Taoist saints, other saints, buddhas,
  bodhisattvas, and all kinds of spiritual fathers and mothers,
Please forgive my ancestors and me for all of the mistakes that we
  have made in all lifetimes.
Please remove soul mind body blockages from my spiritual, mental,
  emotional, and physical bodies, from head to toe, skin to bone.
In order to be forgiven I will serve unconditionally.
To chant, meditate, and offer all kinds of acts of kindness, including
  love, forgiveness, compassion, light, generosity, sincerity, honesty,
  and more, are important services to offer humanity.
I will offer these services a lot.
Thank you. Thank you. Thank you.

Mind Power. Visualize golden light radiating in the area of your Ming Men acupuncture point and spreading throughout your whole body, from head to toe, skin to bone, as you chant.

Sound Power. Chant silently or aloud:

> *Tao Love, Tao Forgiveness, Tao Compassion, Tao Light priceless*
> *treasures heal my spiritual, mental, emotional, and physical*
> *bodies. I cannot thank you enough.*
> *Tao Love, Tao Forgiveness, Tao Compassion, Tao Light priceless*
> *treasures heal my spiritual, mental, emotional, and physical*
> *bodies. I cannot thank you enough.*
> *Tao Love, Tao Forgiveness, Tao Compassion, Tao Light priceless*
> *treasures heal my spiritual, mental, emotional, and physical*
> *bodies. I cannot thank you enough.*
> *Tao Love, Tao Forgiveness, Tao Compassion, Tao Light priceless*
> *treasures heal my spiritual, mental, emotional, and physical*
> *bodies. I cannot thank you enough…*

Stop reading. Continue to practice and chant for ten minutes. Remember, for chronic or life-threatening conditions chant two hours or more per day. The more often you chant and the longer you chant, the better. Chant these four sacred and phenomenal treasures silently all of the time to keep them activated. They are unconditional servants always ready to give you healing and blessing. We cannot imagine how much healing and blessing we can receive. We truly cannot honor the Tao Source's generosity enough for giving these treasures to every reader. The Source is giving humanity unconditional service, which is selfless service. Humanity is extremely honored and blessed.

Practice. Practice. Practice.

Benefit. Benefit. Benefit.

My physical life and soul journey have been saved

I am an incredibly blessed person. My physical life and soul journey have been saved by our dear Master Sha many times. Without these interventions I would not be here today to serve Master Sha's mission and complete my tasks here on Mother Earth

I have had serious, chronic physical challenges: asthma, blockages in the respiratory system, and Crohn's disease, which has manifested in my lower abdominal area. Both of these conditions have caused me much pain and were intended, as the manifestation of my karma, to shorten my life.

When I met Master Sha in 2003 I learned how to do self-healing. I also began to receive Divine Karma Cleansing and Divine Downloads to help me even more. For long periods of time I didn't suffer any symptoms at all. I also knew, though, that I had higher levels of karma that could manifest at any time.

In the last two years that has happened.

These karmic attacks were swift. There was no gradual build-up and, each time, I was very, very ill within hours. In May 2011 I was virtually bedridden with both Crohn's and respiratory issues. I was in terrible pain in the lower abdomen, everything was blocked, and breathing was very difficult. Master Sha was in Europe at the time, and when he contacted me I knew I was very close to death. It was that quick.

I could feel the qi, the life force, leaving my body. When he called me, I was alone on the floor of my bedroom, crawling to get to the washroom. Knowing that death was near, I had already begun to prepare myself to transition. I knew that it could be my time to leave.

When Master Sha came on the phone, I felt his love and his determination to save my life. There were other Divine Channels with him and they too were offering their love and support. That alone was heart-touching and I was enormously moved. Readings were done and it was clear I was dealing with a huge amount of karma and the dark souls were committed to take my life.

Master Sha cleared the blockages quickly, even though there was great resistance from the dark souls. He then gave me many Soul Mind Body Transplants and other treasures to revive my body, but my qi was almost gone. He then gave me—from his own being—the life force from his Jin Dan. I then began to rally. I had been lying still on the floor and now was able to sit up. Others who heard me on the telephone said that my voice changed and I sounded alive. This was truly miraculous.

I realized immediately how much Master Sha had to give of himself in order for me to survive. Even now, as I write this, I can feel the tears coming. Master Sha saved my life at the risk of his own. This is how great his love is.

I not only survived, but recovered completely within a few weeks.

As if this were not enough, an almost identical situation occurred less than a year ago. I suffered a major karmic attack that came on with incredible speed. Master Sha was teaching a Soul Language workshop at the Toronto Love Peace Harmony Centre in the fall of 2012. On Friday I was there and everything was fine. On Saturday I awoke in terrible pain, and by the afternoon, I was bedridden and experiencing the same blockages I had encountered in 2011. This time the qi was leaving me even more quickly and I couldn't move at all. I felt that I was dying. My sister came to my house to check on me and I was so pale and so still that she thought I had already transitioned.

Master Sha also dealt with this high-level karma remotely, cleared the blockages, and with many people worldwide listening on the phone, again shared his Jin Dan with me so I could live. He also gave me jing (matter) and qi (energy) to bring my body back as it was still weak and damaged. This time the Heaven's Generals that came to clear the karma were attacked ferociously and many lost their lives. I could see this. Their sacrifice and Master Sha's willingness to give his own life force touched me beyond words. Again, as I write this, the tears are coming. I recovered again within days.

I have described two instances when my life has been saved by the intervention of Master Sha. These were truly miracle healings. I was almost gone and preparing for death. My oil lamp was less than 5% full both times. I know that I am here only because of Master Sha's love and his total commitment to serve humanity and all souls at this time.

I can only vow to do the same.

Thank you. Thank you. Thank you.

Master Lynne Nusyna
Toronto, Canada

Divine Karma Cleansing shrinks brain tumor

In May 2012 I started having trouble lifting my right leg. I went to several doctors who treated me for my hip and spine, giving me medicine and physical therapy, but there was no improvement. By August 2012 it had gotten to a point where I could not lift my left leg and I was having trouble using my right arm. The doctors suspected I had a stroke and were going to treat me as such.

Master Sha was coming to Hilo, Hawaii in the middle of August, so I made an appointment for a private consultation with him. Master Sha told me, "In my spiritual finding, you may have a brain tumor. If not treated, it could seriously affect your life in two years." He advised me to consult a physician as soon as possible. Master Sha then gave me Divine Karma Cleansing and Soul Mind Body Transplants for my major organs and to assist in recovery from my brain tumor.

Arriving back in Honolulu, I contacted a neurologist, who immediately arranged for me to have an MRI. The results confirmed that I had a brain tumor that had to be removed right away or the doctors said I would lose my life in two years or less. The tumor was on the left side of my brain and somewhat embedded in the brain. The doctors said they would try to get as much of the tumor out as they could, but recovery would be at the most 80%, and it would be a long process. I continued chanting as Master Sha instructed.

When the operation was done, the doctors said that the tumor had reduced to a point of just sitting on my brain, and all they had to do was literally scoop it out. My recovery was amazing: I was 96% recovered within two months—all of this because of Master Sha and the Divine!

Thank you. Thank you. Thank you.

Patrick Sambueno, Sr.
Hawaii, U.S.A.

Tao (Source) Soul Operation

Conventional modern medicine uses surgery to remove matter blockages and to restore function. Nearly two thousand years ago, Hua Tuo, a renowned doctor of traditional Chinese medicine in history, performed the first surgery in China using anesthesia with herbs and wine.

Conventional medicine uses special instruments to open an area of the body for surgery. Tao (Source) Soul Operation means that The Source performs a *spiritual* operation. The Source sends light to an area of the body. The light will open the area spiritually, from skin to bone, and clear soul mind body blockages from the requested area. The area is then closed with Source light sutures and smoothed over.

The Divine and Tao gave me the honor to create hundreds of Divine Soul Operation Master Healers on Mother Earth. Together they have created thousands of soul healing miracles. I will share a few soul healing miracle stories that have been created by Soul Operations.

Divine Soul Operation clears blockage in throat

On Monday, August 26, 2013 I received a life-saving blessing for my heart from Master Sha. That morning I awoke feeling tired, with the beginning of a migraine, no appetite, and a little bit of pressure in my chest. As I drank some tea, I felt a now-familiar constriction in the middle of my chest and realized that my heart was once again challenged. My only thought was "karma!"

As I walked to work, my body felt heavy and my breathing was strained. Every bone and muscle in my back and shoulders hurt. An hour later, the world was beginning to feel like it was moving in slow motion and the pressure in my chest had become uncomfortable. Within another hour, I received The Source Order for Da Tao Mi Zhou for the Heart through Master Sha.

Very, very heavy darkness (karma) was instantly removed, and the pressure in my chest and the pain in my physical heart and back subsided. In an instant, my whole body felt clear and I could breathe again. According to the soul reading I received, the karma was so very heavy that I could have had a fatal heart attack in less than twenty-four hours.

Until six weeks ago, I have not been aware of or experienced heart issues. Six weeks ago, I experienced constriction in my chest. Within minutes of finishing a two-hour practice, as I took a bite of food, I felt a blockage in the middle of my chest at the level of the sternum. My throat was open so I could swallow, but the food struggled through the constricted pathway. I began to feel faint and scanned the kitchen for the phone, but realized that I could not reach it. Instantly, I was guided to offer myself a Divine Soul Operation. Within seconds, the blockage cleared. No pain. No gasping. Just a clear and open passage.

Gratitude towards Master Sha filled my soul, heart, mind, and body. Thank you for transmitting this powerful healing treasure to me. Thank you for opening my spiritual channels so I could receive the message to apply this priceless divine treasure. At that moment, I did not know that the Soul Operation had saved my life. I was simply overflowing with deep gratitude for Master Sha; grateful that he had guided me and so many others to receive this healing treasure. "Thank you" will never be enough.

I am extremely blessed and grateful. Through Master Sha I have learned to self-heal and to help others heal. It is my hope that you will be inspired to apply soul healing to transform your health, relationships, finances, and business and, in the process, may you experience inner joy, inner peace, and fulfill your soul's purpose.

Service to humanity is the only way I can express my deep gratitude to you, the Divine, Tao, and The Source for all I have received. Countless bowdowns.

X. G.
San Francisco, California, U.S.A.

Glucose level drops forty-two points in nineteen minutes

During the Source Soul Operation that I received remotely by webcast, I requested healing for my pancreas as I have been having elevated blood glucose levels.

Immediately after the Soul Operation I checked my level and the reading was 131. I continued to focus on the pancreas during the chanting that followed. I retested and got a reading of 89! This was 19 minutes after the first reading.

Thank you, Master Sha, the Divine, Tao, and Source.

S. W. K.
Kentucky, U.S.A

One Divine Soul Operation heals severe anxiety

Eight years ago I began to suffer from anxiety. I would awaken every night with an anxiety attack. I tried various healing modalities and herbs and still I suffered. Nothing helped. Months before, I had read a book by a renowned healer, TCM doctor, and spiritual master who was also a grandmaster of many ancient disciplines. That extraordinary being was Dr. and Master Sha. I learned that he was holding a workshop near my home, and I went. On the very first day of the workshop, Dr. and Master Sha offered everyone a Divine Soul Operation for one request. I requested healing of my emotions.

Something shifted in those few minutes, and my life has never been the same. From that day—eight years ago—up to now—I have never experienced another anxiety attack. Not even once! My life was transformed by this blessing and further transformed by many blessings, teachings, and treasures I have received since.

Since that day, I have studied soul healing, wisdom, and practices to transform health, emotions, relationships, and every aspect of life. I have become a Divine Healer and am empowered to offer healing to my loved ones, others, and myself. I enthusiastically share soul healing techniques and practices with others because I know they can be helped with these simple and very powerful methods for self-healing and transformation.

I am deeply honored to be a student of Dr. and Master Sha, who has dedicated his life to serving others and bringing healing, enlightenment, and love, peace, and harmony to humanity and all souls. I cannot honor and thank Master Sha, the Divine, Tao, Source, and all of Heaven enough.

C. E.
Missouri, U.S.A.

Now I am going to offer a one-time Tao Source Soul Operation for every reader. Just remember, this is a one-time Tao Source Soul Operation offering. Please do not ask for a second Soul Operation.

The Source has pre-programmed the Soul Operation within this book for you to receive once and only once for two minutes of healing. You may receive great results, as in the above stories. You may feel a little better. You may feel no change. Everyone responds differently. At the soul level, every reader will receive some benefits. Soul mind body blockages will be partially removed. Some of you could feel better instantly, others tomorrow, and still others one or two weeks later.

I have trained hundreds of Soul Operation Master Healers worldwide. All of my Worldwide Representatives, who are also Divine Channels, can offer a Divine Soul Operation.

Be aware of the time. This silent pre-programmed Soul Operation will last for two minutes only.

I have asked The Source to pre-program the power in this book.

Totally relax. Now it is time for you to be quiet and to receive two minutes of Source Soul Operation.

Prepare! Sit up straight. Put both palms on your lower abdomen below the navel.

Then say the following:

> *I am very honored to receive the pre-programmed Source Soul*
> *   Operation from Dr. and Master Sha.*
> *Please heal my _____* (name the organ, system, part of the
>   body, or condition that needs healing).
> *Thank you.*

Choose one system, organ, part of the body, or health condition and say:

> *I am ready to receive the Source pre-programmed Soul Operation for*
> *   a one-time healing.*
> *Thank you.*
> *Please start.*

Then close your eyes for two minutes to receive the Source Soul Operation.

After two minutes, please offer gratitude by saying *Thank you.*

All readers can receive the pre-programmed Soul Operation healing only once. You may need more than one Soul Operation to continue to clear soul mind body blockages for your request. If you want to receive more Soul Operations, any Divine Channel or Divine Soul Operation Master Healer worldwide would be delighted to serve you.

Tao (Source) Soul Herbs

Healing with Chinese herbs is one of the most important and widely-used treatments of traditional Chinese medicine. The herbs of trad-itional Chinese medicine have served millions of people in the last five thousand years. Today, Chinese herbs are popular worldwide. They are used in almost every country. There are also Indian herbs, indigenous peoples' herbs, and many others. Almost every country and every culture has its own herbs and medicinal plants for treating sickness.

What I am offering is not physical herbs; I am offering Soul Herbs. What does this mean? Remember the teaching: everyone and everything has a soul. This means that every herb has a soul. The Divine and Tao gave me the honor and authority to offer Divine and Tao Soul Herbs downloads. There are herb gardens on Mother Earth. There are also herb gardens in different realms of Heaven and Tao. Divine and Tao herbs may not exist on Mother Earth.

In 2003 the Divine gave me the honor and authority to transmit Divine Soul Herbs from the Divine's Soul Herbs Garden to humanity. The Divine Soul Herbs offer divine herbs in *soul form* from Heaven to the recipient. Tao Source Soul Herbs offer The Source herbs in *soul form* from Heaven to the recipient.

"Soul form" means *light being*. Every Soul Herb is a light being with a different size, shape, and appearance.

Now I am going to offer a Tao Source Soul Herbs Formula for one system, organ, part of the body, or health condition of your choice as a gift. This is a one-time offer. This means you can make a request only one time for one bodily system, organ, part of the body, or health condition.

Prepare! Sit up straight. Put both palms below the navel on your lower abdomen. Silently invoke:

> *Dear Master Sha's pre-programmed Soul Herbs with Tao Source,*
> *I love you, honor you, and appreciate you.*
> *Please give me a soul transmission of Soul Herbs for* _____ (name
>   one system or one organ or one part of the body or one health
>   condition).
> *Thank you.*

Prepare! Tao Source has already prepared one Soul Herbs Formula for you. You will not be able to make a second request.

Tao Source Soul Herbs for One System or One Organ or One Part of the Body or One Health Condition

Transmission!

Congratulations! You are extremely blessed.

This is a Soul Herbs Formula specially created by Heaven to serve your request. You can use the Soul Herbs treasures anytime, anywhere.

This is how to apply them:

> *Dear Tao Source Soul Herbs,*
> *I love you and honor you.*
> *Please turn on to heal me.*
> *I am very grateful.*
> *Thank you.*

Then chant:

> *Tao Source Soul Herbs heal me. Thank you.*
> *Tao Source Soul Herbs heal me. Thank you.*
> *Tao Source Soul Herbs heal me. Thank you.*
> *Tao Source Soul Herbs heal me. Thank you...*

Stop reading. Chant for ten minutes. As with all soul treasures you have received, for chronic or life-threatening conditions, chant two hours or more per day. You can add all of your practice time together to total at least two hours per day. In fact, there is no time limit. The more you chant, the more healing benefits you could receive.

Slipped disc surgery canceled after one Soul Herbs blessing

In September 2004 I attended my first retreat with Master Sha, a Body Space Medicine Retreat at Asilomar in Pacific Grove, California. In addition to the great teachings, I received a permanent download (transmission) of forty-two Soul Herbs that I can apply to offer healing blessings to others.

Two months later Master Sha conducted a two-day Introductory Body Space Medicine workshop in Toronto. The event was also transmitted via teleconference and live webcast to students all over North America.

Since I was the only person in Toronto who had received the Soul Herbs treasures, I was asked by Master Sha on the second day to offer soul healing blessings to participants who had pain, whether they were present in person or participating via teleconference and webcast. A dozen people came forward with varying degrees of pain in different parts of the body. They were asked to describe their pain before they received the Soul Herbs healing blessing. Some had knee pain, some back pain, etc. I invoked my Soul Herbs treasures and offered soul healing blessings to everyone on stage and to those on the teleconference and webcast who had made a request. The blessing lasted no more than three minutes.

Following the blessing, everyone was asked to share their experience, and all had positive responses, including a lady with back pain who shared that her pain was significantly reduced. People on the live call and webcast also reported positive results, including a person from Hawaii and another from Illinois.

About two weeks later at a Learning Annex workshop led by Master Sha, a student approached Master Sha and asked if he remembered a friend of hers who attended the two-day workshop where the Soul Herbs blessing was given. She shared that her friend had experienced tremendous healing for her slipped discs, which had been giving her a lot of pain. After the Soul Herbs blessing, she felt so good and had so little pain that she cancelled her previously scheduled slipped disc surgery. Furthermore, sometime later this student reported that her friend had planned to cancel her travel abroad due to her back issues but ended up going as she no longer had back pain.

Thank you, Master Sha for these tremendous treasures, which I still use very often.

Robert L.
North York, Ontario, Canada

There are so many Divine and Tao treasures. In one sentence:

**What we have on Mother Earth is what soul treasures
the Divine and Tao have in Heaven.**

I am extremely grateful to be a servant of humanity and all souls, as well as a Divine and Tao servant, vehicle, and channel. I am extremely honored to have trained and certified more than thirty Divine Channels. I am extremely honored to be training nearly four hundred Divine Channels-in-Training throughout the world. Within two or three years, there could be hundreds of Divine Channels on Mother Earth. All Divine Channels are given the honor and authority to offer permanent divine treasures to humanity.

This is the first time in history that the Divine and Tao have given so many people the authority and honor to offer Heaven's treasures from the Divine and Tao.

People speak about Heaven coming to Mother Earth. Divine and Tao treasures are the highest gifts of Heaven coming to Mother Earth. When one receives a Divine or Tao treasure, including Soul Herbs, Soul Mind Body Transplants, and many more, one receives and carries Divine and Tao presence in a very powerful way.

Thank you, the Divine.
Thank you, Tao.
Love you, the Divine.
Love you, Tao.
We are extremely honored.
We are extremely blessed.

3

Sacred Source Jin Dan Meditation for Healing, Rejuvenation, Prolonging Life, and Transforming Relationships, Finances, and Every Aspect of Life

WHEN I AWOKE early on August 7, 2013, The Source taught me a sacred and very powerful meditation to develop energy, stamina, vitality, and immunity; to rejuvenate and prolong life; and to move in the direction of immortality. I was so honored to receive this teaching from The Source to share with humanity.

August 7, 2013 was a very special day. At this moment it is 10:30 p.m. Eastern Daylight Time on August 8, 2013. Today is the tenth birthday of the Soul Light Era. In this chapter I am flowing the sacred meditation that The Source gave to me yesterday morning.

Before I share this sacred meditation, I will offer some foundation teaching so that you can understand the key sacred wisdom of the meditation.

I will start with the Jin Dan.

What Is the Jin Dan?

"Jin" means *gold*. "Dan" means *light ball*. "Jin Dan" means *golden light ball*. The Jin Dan is located in the lower abdomen, just below the navel in the center of the body. No one is born with a Jin Dan. It requires special spiritual practice to create a Jin Dan.

A Jin Dan is made of jing qi shen. A human being's jing qi shen is not enough to form a Jin Dan. The jing qi shen of Heaven and Mother Earth is needed to form a Jin Dan. From ancient times up to now, serious spiritual practitioners have practiced dedicatedly for two hours or more a day for a minimum of thirty years to form a Jin Dan the size of a fist.

The Power and Significance of the Jin Dan

- Jin Dan is the key to boosting energy, stamina, vitality, and immunity.
- Jin Dan is the key to healing the spiritual, mental, emotional, and physical bodies.
- Jin Dan is the key to preventing all sickness.
- Jin Dan is the key to rejuvenating the soul, heart, mind, and body.
- Jin Dan is the key to prolonging life.
- Jin Dan is the key to moving in the direction of immortality.
- Jin Dan is the key to opening spiritual channels.
- Jin Dan is the key to developing the intelligence of the mind, heart, and soul.
- Jin Dan is the key for enlightening soul, mind, and body.
- Jin Dan is the key to transforming relationships.
- Jin Dan is the key to transforming finances and business.
- Jin Dan is the key to offering service to others.

From the above points it is not difficult for every reader to realize that the Jin Dan is the key sacred treasure to transform all life. How does it work? Please study my books *Tao I*, *Tao II*, and *Tao Song and Tao Dance* for Jin Dan teachings. In one sentence:

Jin Dan is the Oneness Ball that is the greatest treasure for all life.

Now let me introduce the Sacred Source Jin Dan Meditation. Read it first. Then I will give you the shorter practical version for your meditation.

Sacred Source Jin Dan Meditation

The purpose of the Sacred Source Jin Dan Meditation is to grow and develop a Jin Dan in a special sacred area of the body. As this Jin Dan grows and develops, all the benefits of boosting energy, healing, preventing sickness, rejuvenation, prolonging life, opening spiritual channels, developing intelligence, enlightening soul, heart, mind, and body, transforming relationships, transforming finances and business, and more can be gained. Every aspect of your life could be blessed.

To save you weeks, months, and years of special practice, The Source will give you an extraordinary permanent treasure of a Jin Dan Seed in this special sacred area of the body. When you understand the power and significance of this gift, you will deeply understand that the generosity of the Divine, Tao, and The Source cannot be expressed in words, comprehended by thoughts, or imagined in any universe. You are extremely blessed. We are all extremely blessed.

Special Sacred Area: Ming Men Acupuncture Point

What is the special sacred area of the body for you to receive a Jin Dan seed and develop a Jin Dan? It is the area of the Ming Men acupuncture point.

"Ming" means *life*. "Men" means *gate*. "Ming Men" means *life gate*. The Ming Men acupuncture point is located on the back opposite and directly behind the navel. (See figure 8 on page 54.)

The Power and Significance of the Ming Men Acupuncture Point

The Ming Men acupuncture point is:

- the "life gate"
- the headquarters of Ming Men fire and Ming Men water
  - Ming Men fire is the most important yang in the body. In addition:

- ◆ Ming Men fire is the root yang of the whole body. It carries the original force of one's life activities. It warms and promotes the physiological functions of all systems and organs.
- ◆ Ming Men fire is the root force for promoting a human being's growth, development, and reproduction.
- ◆ Ming Men fire promotes water metabolism.
  - ○ Ming Men water is the most important yin in the body. In addition:
    - ◆ Ming Men water is the material foundation of the kidney yang function.
    - ◆ Ming Men water nourishes all systems and organs.
- • the hub of the most important energy circle and the most important matter circle
  - ○ The most important energy circle starts from the Hui Yin (pronounced *hway yeen*) acupuncture point on the perineum, between the genitals and anus. It flows up through the seven Soul Houses or energy chakras to the Bai Hui acupuncture point (pronounced *bye hway*) at the top of the head. From there, it flows down through the Wai Jiao[13] (pronounced *wye jee-yow*), which is the biggest space in the body, and finally back to the Hui Yin acupuncture point. See figure 10 on page 58.
    - ◆ This most important energy circle is the key for healing all sickness in the spiritual, mental, emotional, and physical bodies.
  - ○ The most important matter circle starts from the Hui Yin acupuncture point between the genitals and anus. From there, it flows to the tailbone, which has an invisible hole. Energy and tiny matter go through this invisible hole and move up through the center of the spinal cord to the brain, and then up to the Bai Hui acupuncture point at the top of the head. From

---

[13] The Wai Jiao was discovered in China by my spiritual mentor and father, Dr. and Master Zhi Chen Guo, after nearly fifty years of clinical research and practice with thousands of patients. The Wai Jiao is located in front of the spinal column and back ribs. It also extends up into the head. It is the biggest space inside the body.

there they go down through the seven Soul Houses or energy chakras back to the Hui Yin acupuncture point. See figure 11 on page 62.

♦ This most important matter circle is the key for rejuvenation, prolonging life, and moving in the direction of immortality.

- **the Tao point**. This is the most important aspect of the Ming Men acupuncture point.
    ○ Tao is the Source.
    ○ Tao is The Way of all life.
    ○ Tao is the universal principles and laws.

In one sentence:

**The Ming Men acupuncture point is the Tao point
to transform all life of a being.**

The Source has released the sacred Xiu Lian meditation in this chapter for the first time. "Xiu" (pronounced *sheo*) means *purification of soul, heart, mind, and body.* "Lian" (pronounced *lyen*) means *practice.* "Xiu Lian" means *purification practice of the soul, heart, mind, and body.* Xiu Lian is the totality of one's spiritual journey. This sacred meditation will benefit the totality of your spiritual journey.

I have explained the sacredness and significance of the Ming Men acupuncture point. Now let me lead you to start the Sacred Source Jin Dan Meditation:

Body Power. Sit up straight with your back free and clear. Place the tip of your tongue gently against the roof of your mouth. Place one palm over your navel and the other palm over your Ming Men acupuncture point.

Soul Power. Say *hello* to inner souls:

Dear soul mind body of my Ming Men acupuncture point,
I love you, honor you, and appreciate you.
You are the key for boosting energy, stamina, vitality, and immunity.

You are the key for healing and rejuvenation.
You are the key to transform all life.
I cannot honor you enough.
Please develop yourself and heal and rejuvenate me.
Thank you.

Say *hello* to outer souls:

Dear Divine,
Dear Tao, The Source,
I love you, honor you, and appreciate you.
Please forgive my ancestors and me for all of our mistakes in all our
*   lifetimes.*
Please remove soul mind body blockages in the Ming Men
*   acupuncture point.*
I am extremely grateful.
Thank you.

Mind Power. Concentrate on the Ming Men acupuncture point on your back directly behind your navel. Visualize a bright golden light point forming in your Ming Men acupuncture point. This golden light is formed from the jing qi shen of your body, of Mother Earth, and of Heaven.

Sound Power. Jing is matter. Qi is energy. Shen is soul. Shen Qi Jing He Yi (pronounced *shun chee jing huh yee*) means *soul, energy, and matter join as one.*

Chant:

Ming Men Shen Qi Jing He Yi to form Ming Men Jin Dan.
Ming Men Shen Qi Jing He Yi to form Ming Men Jin Dan.
Ming Men Shen Qi Jing He Yi to form Ming Men Jin Dan.
Ming Men Shen Qi Jing He Yi to form Ming Men Jin Dan.
Ming Men Shen Qi Jing He Yi to form Ming Men Jin Dan.
Ming Men Shen Qi Jing He Yi to form Ming Men Jin Dan.
Ming Men Shen Qi Jing He Yi to form Ming Men Jin Dan . . .

Chant and visualize for about five minutes. If your Third Eye is open you could see a light spot in the area of your Ming Men acupuncture point. If your Third Eye is not open, imagine a golden light spot forming there. To form this Ming Men Jin Dan by yourself would take a long, long time by doing this practice and other secret, sacred practices very dedicatedly. I have an extraordinary sacred way to help you to form your Ming Men Jin Dan.

Step 1. Receive The Source Ming Men Jin Dan Seed

The initial size of the Ming Men Jin Dan is about ten percent of the size of a grain of rice. It is like a seed. This Ming Men Jin Dan is highly concentrated jing qi shen of your body, Mother Earth, and Heaven joined as one.

A human being's jing qi shen is not enough to form this Ming Men Jin Dan. This is the first time in history that The Source has released this sacred way to form the Ming Men Jin Dan. The Ming Men Jin Dan must be formed by gathering the jing qi shen of Tian Di Ren. "Tian" means *Heaven*. "Di" means *Mother Earth*. "Ren" means *human being*. "Tian Di Ren" (pronounced *tyen dee wren*) means *Heaven, Mother Earth, human being*.

Ancient spiritual practice has used secret, sacred chants and visualizations that must be practiced at specific times of the day to form this Ming Men Jin Dan. As I explained earlier, a spiritual practitioner could take a long, long time to create even an initial small seed of a Jin Dan. But the traditional way does not create this initial Jin Dan in the area of the Ming Men acupuncture point.

I am extremely honored to be a servant and vehicle of the Divine and Tao. I have received the honor and authority to offer their permanent priceless Soul Mind Body Transplants since July 2003.

I can serve you and all readers by offering a Source Ming Men Jin Dan Seed to you through a pre-programed Order from The Source. Prepare to receive this honor and priceless permanent treasure for healing, rejuvenation, longevity, and transforming relationships, finances, and every aspect of life. Totally relax. Open your heart and soul. Be very grateful that you can receive this extraordinary treasure from The Source.

Countless beloved buddhas, holy saints, healing angels, and all kinds of spiritual fathers and mothers have not received this honor.

Now I am extremely honored and happy to serve you and every reader to receive a seed of Ming Men Jin Dan as a gift from the Divine, Tao, and my heart.

Prepare! Sit up straight. Close your eyes. Totally relax. Put both palms on your lower abdomen.

**The Source Order: Ming Men Jin Dan Seed
Soul Mind Body Transplants**

Transmission!

Congratulations! You are extremely blessed.

Thank you, the Divine, Tao, and The Source for your generosity to offer these priceless permanent treasures as a gift to every reader.

After receiving this treasure, you and every reader have the seed of a Ming Men Jin Dan. This Ming Men Jin Dan Seed is about ten percent of the size of a grain of rice. The more you practice, the more the Jin Dan will grow in size.

Continue to practice. Visualize this Ming Men Jin Dan Seed rotating counterclockwise. At the same time, silently chant:

> *The Source Ming Men Jin Dan Seed is shining, vibrating, and
>   rotating counterclockwise. Thank you.*
> *The jing qi shen of The Source and Tian Di Ren He Yi grow my Ming
>   Men Jin Dan. Thank you.*
> *The Source Ming Men Jin Dan Seed is shining, vibrating, and
>   rotating counterclockwise. Thank you.*
> *The jing qi shen of The Source and Tian Di Ren He Yi grow my Ming
>   Men Jin Dan. Thank you.*
> *The Source Ming Men Jin Dan Seed is shining, vibrating, and
>   rotating counterclockwise. Thank you.*
> *The jing qi shen of The Source and Tian Di Ren He Yi grow my Ming
>   Men Jin Dan. Thank you.*

*The Source Ming Men Jin Dan Seed is shining, vibrating, and
    rotating counterclockwise. Thank you.*
*The jing qi shen of The Source and Tian Di Ren He Yi grow my Ming
    Men Jin Dan. Thank you.*
*The Source Ming Men Jin Dan Seed is shining, vibrating, and
    rotating counterclockwise. Thank you.*
*The jing qi shen of The Source and Tian Di Ren He Yi grow my Ming
    Men Jin Dan. Thank you.*
*The Source Ming Men Jin Dan Seed is shining, vibrating, and
    rotating counterclockwise. Thank you.*
*The jing qi shen of The Source and Tian Di Ren He Yi grow my Ming
    Men Jin Dan. Thank you.*
*The Source Ming Men Jin Dan Seed is shining, vibrating, and
    rotating counterclockwise. Thank you.*
*The jing qi shen of The Source and Tian Di Ren He Yi grow my Ming
    Men Jin Dan. Thank you...*

Practice for five minutes.
Now visualize the Ming Men Jin Dan growing to the size of your fist.
Continue to visualize and chant for five minutes more:

*The Source Ming Men Jin Dan Seed is shining, vibrating, and
    rotating counterclockwise. Thank you.*
*The jing qi shen of The Source and Tian Di Ren He Yi grow my Ming
    Men Jin Dan. Thank you...*

Then the Jin Dan expands to the size of your lower abdomen.
Visualize the Jin Dan rotating counterclockwise and chant for another
five minutes:

*The Source Ming Men Jin Dan Seed is shining, vibrating, and
    rotating counterclockwise. Thank you.*
*The jing qi shen of The Source and Tian Di Ren He Yi grow my Ming
    Men Jin Dan. Thank you...*

Then the Jin Dan expands and expands to the size of your whole abdomen. Continue for five minutes to visualize the Ming Men Jin Dan expanded to the size of your whole abdomen, from the diaphragm to the genitals.

At the same time, chant:

> *The Source Ming Men Jin Dan Seed is shining, vibrating, and*
> *rotating counterclockwise. Thank you.*
> *The jing qi shen of The Source and Tian Di Ren He Yi grow my Ming*
> *Men Jin Dan. Thank you…*

Continue to visualize the Jin Dan expanding from the abdomen to fill your entire torso. Chant for five minutes more:

> *The Source Ming Men Jin Dan Seed is shining, vibrating, and*
> *rotating counterclockwise. Thank you.*
> *The jing qi shen of The Source and Tian Di Ren He Yi grow my Ming*
> *Men Jin Dan. Thank you…*

Now let us move to step two.

Step 2. *Visualize Your Ming Men Jin Dan Expanding to the Size of Your Body*

Continue to visualize the Jin Dan expanding to the size of your whole body, from head to toe, skin to bone. Continue to chant and visualize:

> *The Source Ming Men Jin Dan Seed is shining, vibrating, and*
> *rotating counterclockwise. Thank you.*
> *The jing qi shen of The Source and Tian Di Ren He Yi grow my Ming*
> *Men Jin Dan. Thank you…*

Please understand that your Ming Men Jin Dan has not actually expanded to the size of your body. You are doing creative visualization. Every moment that you practice this visualization and chanting, your Jin Dan will expand little by little.

Continue to chant and visualize:

The Source Tian Di Ren Shen Qi Jing He Yi (pronounced tyen dee wren shun chee jing huh yee) expands my Jin Dan. Thank you.
The Source Tian Di Ren Shen Qi Jing He Yi expands my Jin Dan. Thank you.
The Source Tian Di Ren Shen Qi Jing He Yi expands my Jin Dan. Thank you.
The Source Tian Di Ren Shen Qi Jing He Yi expands my Jin Dan. Thank you.
The Source Tian Di Ren Shen Qi Jing He Yi expands my Jin Dan. Thank you.
The Source Tian Di Ren Shen Qi Jing He Yi expands my Jin Dan. Thank you.
The Source Tian Di Ren Shen Qi Jing He Yi expands my Jin Dan. Thank you...

Continue to meditate and visualize the Jin Dan rotating counterclockwise. Your body also rotates counterclockwise with your Jin Dan. Keep your eyes closed. You and your Jin Dan are one.

Chant silently and visualize:

Jin Dan is vibrating, radiating, and growing.
Jin Dan is vibrating, radiating, and growing.
Jin Dan is vibrating, radiating, and growing.
Jin Dan is vibrating, radiating, and growing.
Jin Dan is vibrating, radiating, and growing.
Jin Dan is vibrating, radiating, and growing.
Jin Dan is vibrating, radiating, and growing...

To have a Ming Men Jin Dan the size of your whole body is to reach Tao. In history a few saints have reached Tao. When they reached Tao, their Jin Dan had grown to the size of their whole body. This indicates that they became immortal. It normally takes a serious spiritual master thousands or even millions of lifetimes to form a Jin Dan the size of one's body.

In the Soul Light Era, a serious soul master could reach Tao in one lifetime because The Source and Heaven's Highest Committees are offering permanent Jin Dan Soul Mind Body Transplants. The opportunity is extremely rare.

Chant and practice for another five minutes. Then move to step three.

Step 3. Visualize Your Jin Dan Expanding to the Size of Mother Earth

Now visualize your Jin Dan expanding beyond the size of your body. At the same time, your body expands as the Jin Dan expands.

First visualize your Jin Dan expanding to the size of your home or workplace.

Then chant:

Jin Dan is vibrating, radiating, and growing.
Jin Dan is vibrating, radiating, and growing.
Jin Dan is vibrating, radiating, and growing.
Jin Dan is vibrating, radiating, and growing.
Jin Dan is vibrating, radiating, and growing.
Jin Dan is vibrating, radiating, and growing.
Jin Dan is vibrating, radiating, and growing...

Next visualize your Jin Dan continuing to expand slowly until it grows to the size of your city. Your body also expands at the same time. Your Jin Dan and body are still rotating counterclockwise.

Continue to chant and visualize:

Jin Dan is vibrating, radiating, and growing.
Jin Dan is vibrating, radiating, and growing.
Jin Dan is vibrating, radiating, and growing.
Jin Dan is vibrating, radiating, and growing.
Jin Dan is vibrating, radiating, and growing.
Jin Dan is vibrating, radiating, and growing.
Jin Dan is vibrating, radiating, and growing...

I would like to emphasize to you and every reader that to chant seven times is not enough. At every stage of this Sacred Source Jin Dan Meditation you need to chant much more than seven times. You can chant for a few minutes or even longer at every stage. There is no time limit. The longer you visualize and chant, the better.

Continue to visualize your Jin Dan expanding to the size of your province or state. Visualize your body expanding to the size of your province or state also.

Continue to chant:

Jin Dan is vibrating, radiating, and growing.
Jin Dan is vibrating, radiating, and growing.
Jin Dan is vibrating, radiating, and growing.
Jin Dan is vibrating, radiating, and growing.
Jin Dan is vibrating, radiating, and growing.
Jin Dan is vibrating, radiating, and growing.
Jin Dan is vibrating, radiating, and growing...

Next visualize and expand your Jin Dan and body to the size of your country while chanting *Ren Di Jing Qi Shen He Yi*. "Ren" means *human being*. "Di" means *Mother Earth*. "Jing" means *matter*. "Qi" means *energy*. "Shen" means *soul*. "He Yi" means *join as one*. "Ren Di Jing Qi Shen He Yi" (pronounced *wren dee jing chee shun huh yee*) means *human being, Mother Earth, energy, matter, and soul join as one*.

Now visualize and expand your Jin Dan and body to the size of Mother Earth.

Chant:

Ren Di Jing Qi Shen He Yi grows my Jin Dan.
Ren Di Jing Qi Shen He Yi grows my Jin Dan.
Ren Di Jing Qi Shen He Yi grows my Jin Dan.
Ren Di Jing Qi Shen He Yi grows my Jin Dan.
Ren Di Jing Qi Shen He Yi grows my Jin Dan.
Ren Di Jing Qi Shen He Yi grows my Jin Dan.
Ren Di Jing Qi Shen He Yi grows my Jin Dan...

Continue to visualize your Jin Dan and body to be the size of Mother Earth. Your Jin Dan and body continue to rotate together. Now chant *Di Jing Hua Zi Yang*. "Di" means *Mother Earth*. "Jing Hua" means *essence, including Mother Earth's soul fruits, vitamins, minerals, amino acids, proteins, nectars, elixirs, and other essential nutrients.* "Zi Yang" means *nourish.* "Di Jing Hua Zi Yang" (pronounced *dee jing hwah dz yahng*) means *the essence of Mother Earth nourishes my Jin Dan.*

Chant *Di Jing Hua Zi Yang* for five minutes:

> *Di Jing Hua Zi Yang grows my Jin Dan. Thank you.*
> *Di Jing Hua Zi Yang grows my Jin Dan. Thank you.*
> *Di Jing Hua Zi Yang grows my Jin Dan. Thank you.*
> *Di Jing Hua Zi Yang grows my Jin Dan. Thank you.*
> *Di Jing Hua Zi Yang grows my Jin Dan. Thank you.*
> *Di Jing Hua Zi Yang grows my Jin Dan. Thank you.*
> *Di Jing Hua Zi Yang grows my Jin Dan. Thank you...*

You can also chant in English for five minutes:

> *Mother Earth's essence nourishes and grows my Jin Dan. Thank you.*
> *Mother Earth's essence nourishes and grows my Jin Dan. Thank you.*
> *Mother Earth's essence nourishes and grows my Jin Dan. Thank you.*
> *Mother Earth's essence nourishes and grows my Jin Dan. Thank you.*
> *Mother Earth's essence nourishes and grows my Jin Dan. Thank you.*
> *Mother Earth's essence nourishes and grows my Jin Dan. Thank you.*
> *Mother Earth's essence nourishes and grows my Jin Dan. Thank*
> * you...*

Then continue to step four.

Step 4. Visualize Your Jin Dan Expanding to the Size of Heaven

Visualize your Jin Dan and your body continuing to rotate counterclockwise and expanding together up to Heaven. Silently chant *Ren Tian He Yi.* "Ren" means *human being.* "Tian" means *Heaven.* "He Yi" means *join as one.* "Ren Tian He Yi" (pronounced *wren tyen huh yee*) means *human being and Heaven join as one.*

Chant:

> *Ren Tian He Yi grows my Jin Dan.*

Ren Tian He Yi grows my Jin Dan.
Ren Tian He Yi grows my Jin Dan.
Ren Tian He Yi grows my Jin Dan.
Ren Tian He Yi grows my Jin Dan.
Ren Tian He Yi grows my Jin Dan.
Ren Tian He Yi grows my Jin Dan…

Jing Qi Shen of Ren Tian join as one to grow my Jin Dan. Thank you.
Jing Qi Shen of Ren Tian join as one to grow my Jin Dan. Thank you.
Jing Qi Shen of Ren Tian join as one to grow my Jin Dan. Thank you.
Jing Qi Shen of Ren Tian join as one to grow my Jin Dan. Thank you.
Jing Qi Shen of Ren Tian join as one to grow my Jin Dan. Thank you.
Jing Qi Shen of Ren Tian join as one to grow my Jin Dan. Thank you.
Jing Qi Shen of Ren Tian join as one to grow my Jin Dan. Thank
    you…

Continue to chant for five minutes.

Your Jin Dan and body are now the size of Heaven. Chant *Tian Jing Hua Zi Yang.* "Tian" means *Heaven.* "Jing Hua" means *essence, including Heaven's soul fruits, vitamins, minerals, amino acids, proteins, nectars, elixirs, and other essential nutrients.* "Zi Yang" means *nourish.* "Tian Jing Hua Zi Yang" (pronounced *tyen jing hwah dz yahng*) means *the essence of Heaven nourishes my Jin Dan.*

Chant *Tian Jing Hua Zi Yang* and meditate for five minutes:

Tian Jing Hua Zi Yang grows my Jin Dan. Thank you.
Tian Jing Hua Zi Yang grows my Jin Dan. Thank you.
Tian Jing Hua Zi Yang grows my Jin Dan. Thank you.
Tian Jing Hua Zi Yang grows my Jin Dan. Thank you.
Tian Jing Hua Zi Yang grows my Jin Dan. Thank you.
Tian Jing Hua Zi Yang grows my Jin Dan. Thank you.
Tian Jing Hua Zi Yang grows my Jin Dan. Thank you…

Now continue to step five.

Step 5. *Visualize Your Jin Dan Expanding to Tao*

Now visualize your Jin Dan and your body expanding to infinity, which is Tao. Continue to imagine your Jin Dan and body rotating counterclockwise. Silently chant *Ren Tao He Yi*. "Ren" means *human being*. "Tao" means *The Source* and *the Creator of Heaven, Mother Earth, and countless planets, stars, galaxies, and universes*. "He Yi" means *join as one*. "Ren Tao He Yi" (pronounced *wren dow huh yee*) means *human being and Tao join as one*.

Chant and visualize:

> *Ren Tao He Yi*
> *Ren Tao He Yi*
> *Ren Tao He Yi*
> *Ren Tao He Yi*
> *Ren Tao He Yi*
> *Ren Tao He Yi*
> *Ren Tao He Yi . . .*

Continue to chant for five minutes.

Your Jin Dan and body are the size of Tao. Now chant *Tao Jing Hua Zi Yang*. "Tao" means *The Source, the Creator*. "Jing Hua" means *essence, including Tao's soul fruits, vitamins, minerals, amino acids, proteins, nectars, elixirs, and other essential nutrients*. "Zi Yang" means *nourish*. "Tao Jing Hua Zi Yang" (pronounced *dow jing hwah dz yahng*) means *the essence of Tao and Heaven nourish my Jin Dan*.

Chant for five minutes:

> *Tao Jing Hua Zi Yang grows my Jin Dan. Thank you.*
> *Tao Jing Hua Zi Yang grows my Jin Dan. Thank you.*
> *Tao Jing Hua Zi Yang grows my Jin Dan. Thank you.*
> *Tao Jing Hua Zi Yang grows my Jin Dan. Thank you.*
> *Tao Jing Hua Zi Yang grows my Jin Dan. Thank you.*
> *Tao Jing Hua Zi Yang grows my Jin Dan. Thank you.*
> *Tao Jing Hua Zi Yang grows my Jin Dan. Thank you . . .*

Tao Ren He Yi (Tao and human being join as one, pronounced
    dow wren huh yee)
Tao Ren He Yi
Tao Ren He Yi
Tao Ren He Yi
Tao Ren He Yi
Tao Ren He Yi
Tao Ren He Yi...

Now your visualization has expanded your Jin Dan and your body
to the size of Tao. Practice five more minutes, and then the meditation
will continue with your Jin Dan and body returning to actual size, one
step at a time.

Step 6. *Visualize Your Jin Dan Returning to the Size of Heaven*

In this step of the sacred practice the Jin Dan will stop rotating counterclockwise and will start to rotate *clockwise*.

Visualize your Jin Dan and body rotating *clockwise* and reducing
together to the size of Heaven.

Chant:

Tao and Tian Jing Qi Shen and Jing Hua (pronounced *dow, tyen jing
    chee shun, jing hwah*) *pour into my body from every direction to
    nourish and grow my true Jin Dan. Thank you.*
*Tao and Tian Jing Qi Shen and Jing Hua pour into my body from
    every direction to nourish and grow my true Jin Dan. Thank you.*
*Tao and Tian Jing Qi Shen and Jing Hua pour into my body from
    every direction to nourish and grow my true Jin Dan. Thank you.*
*Tao and Tian Jing Qi Shen and Jing Hua pour into my body from
    every direction to nourish and grow my true Jin Dan. Thank you.*
*Tao and Tian Jing Qi Shen and Jing Hua pour into my body from
    every direction to nourish and grow my true Jin Dan. Thank you.*
*Tao and Tian Jing Qi Shen and Jing Hua pour into my body from
    every direction to nourish and grow my true Jin Dan. Thank you.*

*Tao and Tian Jing Qi Shen and Jing Hua pour into my body from
every direction to nourish and grow my true Jin Dan. Thank
you...*

Continue to chant and visualize for five minutes. Then move to step
seven.

Step 7. *Visualize Your Jin Dan Returning to the Size of Mother Earth*

Visualize your Jin Dan rotating clockwise and reducing from the size
of Heaven to the size of Mother Earth. At the same time, visualize your
body reducing to the size of Mother Earth.
    Chant:

Tian and Di Jing Qi Shen and Jing Hua (pronounced *tyen, dee jing
chee shun, jing hwah*) *pour into my body from every direction to
nourish and grow my true Jin Dan. Thank you.*

*Tian and Di Jing Qi Shen and Jing Hua pour into my body from every
direction to nourish and grow my true Jin Dan. Thank you.*

*Tian and Di Jing Qi Shen and Jing Hua pour into my body from every
direction to nourish and grow my true Jin Dan. Thank you.*

*Tian and Di Jing Qi Shen and Jing Hua pour into my body from every
direction to nourish and grow my true Jin Dan. Thank you.*

*Tian and Di Jing Qi Shen and Jing Hua pour into my body from every
direction to nourish and grow my true Jin Dan. Thank you.*

*Tian and Di Jing Qi Shen and Jing Hua pour into my body from every
direction to nourish and grow my true Jin Dan. Thank you.*

*Tian and Di Jing Qi Shen and Jing Hua pour into my body from every
direction to nourish and grow my true Jin Dan. Thank you...*

Continue to chant and visualize for five minutes. Then move to step
eight.

Step 8. *Visualize Your Jin Dan Returning to the Size of Your Body*

Visualize your Jin Dan continuing to rotate clockwise and reducing
from the size of Mother Earth to the size of your body.

Chant:

> *Di and Body Jing Qi Shen and Jing Hua (pronounced dee, jing chee shun, jing hwah) pour into my body from every direction to nourish and grow my true Jin Dan. Thank you.*
> *Di and Body Jing Qi Shen and Jing Hua pour into my body from every direction to nourish and grow my true Jin Dan. Thank you.*
> *Di and Body Jing Qi Shen and Jing Hua pour into my body from every direction to nourish and grow my true Jin Dan. Thank you.*
> *Di and Body Jing Qi Shen and Jing Hua pour into my body from every direction to nourish and grow my true Jin Dan. Thank you.*
> *Di and Body Jing Qi Shen and Jing Hua pour into my body from every direction to nourish and grow my true Jin Dan. Thank you.*
> *Di and Body Jing Qi Shen and Jing Hua pour into my body from every direction to nourish and grow my true Jin Dan. Thank you.*
> *Di and Body Jing Qi Shen and Jing Hua pour into my body from every direction to nourish and grow my true Jin Dan. Thank you...*

Continue to chant and visualize for five minutes. Then move to step nine.

Step 9. Visualize Your Jin Dan Returning to the Size of Your Ming Men Acupuncture Point

Visualize your Jin Dan rotating clockwise and reducing from the size of your body to the size of your Ming Men acupuncture point. Your body is now its actual physical size.

Chant and meditate:

> *Tao and Tian Di Ren Jing Qi Shen and Jing Hua (pronounced dow, tyen dee wren jing chee shun, jing hwah) pour into my Ming Men acupuncture point from every direction to nourish and grow my true Jin Dan. Thank you.*
> *Tao and Tian Di Ren Jing Qi Shen and Jing Hua pour into my Ming Men acupuncture point from every direction to nourish and grow my true Jin Dan. Thank you.*

Tao and Tian Di Ren Jing Qi Shen and Jing Hua pour into my Ming
*   Men acupuncture point from every direction to nourish and grow*
*   my true Jin Dan. Thank you.*
Tao and Tian Di Ren Jing Qi Shen and Jing Hua pour into my Ming
*   Men acupuncture point from every direction to nourish and grow*
*   my true Jin Dan. Thank you.*
Tao and Tian Di Ren Jing Qi Shen and Jing Hua pour into my Ming
*   Men acupuncture point from every direction to nourish and grow*
*   my true Jin Dan. Thank you.*
Tao and Tian Di Ren Jing Qi Shen and Jing Hua pour into my Ming
*   Men acupuncture point from every direction to nourish and grow*
*   my true Jin Dan. Thank you.*
Tao and Tian Di Ren Jing Qi Shen and Jing Hua pour into my Ming
*   Men acupuncture point from every direction to nourish and grow*
*   my true Jin Dan. Thank you…*

Continue to chant and visualize for five minutes.

I shared part of this sacred meditation in a teleconference and received very positive feedback from participants. I will share a few stories here, and then summarize this sacred practice.

Source light spread through my being and healed intense pain

Beloved Master Sha,

Thank you for this most sacred wisdom and beautiful light-filled, nourishment-filled chanting practice.

I have received a HUGE healing during the practice. The intense pain that has been with me for over three weeks now feels 90% better. What I saw was that through my tiny Ming Men acupuncture point came in light from the realms of The Source. The light spread through my being and the Ming Men point became the focus like a sun and the rays spread through my body.

My soul feels it has received such upliftment; words cannot express it. Chanting with Master Sha has opened up a gateway for all of us on an enchanting journey. For a few moments we connected with the deepest purity and brightest light. We stepped into a different reality, a reality in which we all became our purest, brightest self. We had a taste of who we were when we were created: light beings.

Master Sha has brought to us the wisdom from The Source. We cannot honor this enough.

Firuzan Mistry
Mumbai, India

Immense power and light

Dear Master Sha,

I am truly speechless by the immense power and magnitude of your teachings and priceless gifts today. I feel so grateful and privileged to have received these teachings of the Sacred Source Ming Men Meditation. I thank you, Tao, and The Source. I still cannot believe my good fortune in having been present.

My entire soul, heart, mind, and body have changed in the last few hours. I feel great energy and stamina but also great balance. My whole body is stronger, especially my lower abdomen and spine. I was filled with light. The heavens opened and immense light and special holy beings filled my house. In fact, the entire universe and I felt merged with the Whole. Everyone receiving this teaching and blessing are joined together, including the countless holy beings who have come for this teaching.

With deepest love and greatest gratitude,

P. S.
California, U.S.A.

Incredible peace and exquisite energy flowed through my body

Dearest Master Sha,

I cannot thank you enough for sharing these new meditation secrets.

The power of focusing on the Ming Men point during sacred chanting and meditation is without equal. I went into the deepest states I have ever experienced and feel incredible peace and exquisite energy flowing through my body. There are surges of energy radiating from the area of my Ming Men point up and down my spine and around my body through all meridians.

The shift in consciousness and insights I have received are too profound for words. I can't wait to immerse myself in this new practice for healing and transformation of physical, mental, emotional, and spiritual health and transformation of relationships, finances, and all aspects of life. This is such a powerful key practice.

Thank you. Thank you. Thank you.

Erik J. Cecil, Esq.
Colorado, U.S.A.

Now I am going to summarize this Sacred Source Jin Dan Meditation. Then you can read and memorize the meditation.

Sacred Source Jin Dan Meditation: Summary

Sit up straight with your feet flat on the floor and your back free and clear. Close your eyes slightly. Place the tip of your tongue gently against the roof of your mouth.

Soul Power. Say *hello*:

> *Dear Divine,*
> *Dear Tao, The Source,*
> *Dear Heaven,*
> *Dear Mother Earth,*
> *Dear countless healing angels, archangels, ascended masters, gurus,*
>   *lamas, kahunas, holy saints, Taoist saints, other saints, buddhas,*
>   *bodhisattvas, and all kinds of spiritual fathers and mothers,*
> *Dear The Source Ling Guang Calligraphy in this book,*[14]
> *Dear my own soul, mind, and body,*
> *I love you, honor you, and appreciate you.*
> *Please help me to develop my Jin Dan to boost my energy, stamina,*
>   *vitality, and immunity; rejuvenate my soul, heart, mind, and body;*

---

[14] Although I have not yet introduced The Source Ling Guang Calligraphy in this book, you can still use Soul Power (Say Hello Healing and Blessing) to invoke and connect with this sacred calligraphy from The Source and request its blessing for your Ming Men Jin Dan.

prolong my life; and transform my relationships, finances, and every aspect of life.
I am very grateful.

Mind Power. Visualize your Ming Men Jin Dan Seed shining bright light in the Ming Men acupuncture point.

Shining. Shining. Shining...
Rotating counterclockwise...
Growing. Growing. Growing.

Sound Power. Chant and visualize together:

The Source Ming Men Jin Dan Seed is shining, vibrating, and rotating counterclockwise. Thank you...

Visualize the Jin Dan expanding to the size of your fist.
Chant and visualize:

Tian Di Ren Shen Qi Jing He Yi (pronounced *tyen dee wren shun chee jing huh yee*) *expands my Jin Dan. Thank you...*

Visualize your Jin Dan continuing to expand to fill your lower abdomen, and then continuing to grow to be as large as your entire torso. Then, visualize the Jin Dan expanding to the size of your body.

Continue to meditate and visualize the Jin Dan rotating *counterclockwise.* Your body also rotates counterclockwise with your Jin Dan. Keep your eyes closed. You and your Jin Dan are one.

Visualize and chant silently:

My Jin Dan is vibrating, resonating, and growing...

Now visualize your Jin Dan expanding beyond the size of your body. At the same time, visualize your body expanding as the Jin Dan expands.

First visualize your Jin Dan and body expanding to the size of your home or workplace.

Chant and visualize:

> *Tian Di Ren Shen Qi Jing He Yi* (pronounced *tyen dee wren shun chee jing huh yee*) *expands my Jin Dan. Thank you...*

Visualize your Jin Dan and body expanding from the size of your home or workplace to the size of your city.
Chant and visualize:

> *Grow my Jin Dan...*

Then continue to chant and visualize:

> *Tian Di Ren Shen Qi Jing He Yi* (pronounced *tyen dee wren shun chee jing huh yee*) *expands my Jin Dan. Thank you...*

Visualize your Jin Dan and body expanding from the size of your city to the size of your province or state.
Chant and visualize:

> *Jin Dan is vibrating and expanding...*

Visualize your Jin Dan and body expanding from the size of your province or state to the size of your country.
Chant and visualize:

> *Shen Qi Jing He Yi* (pronounced *shun chee jing huh yee*) *grows my Jin Dan...*

Visualize your Jin Dan and body expanding from the size of your country to the size of Mother Earth. Your Jin Dan is continually shining and rotating counterclockwise. Your body continues to rotate counterclockwise with your Jin Dan.
Chant and visualize:

> *Mother Earth's Jing Qi Shen nourishes and grows my Jin Dan...*

Visualize your Jin Dan and body expanding from the size of Mother Earth to the size of Heaven.
Chant and visualize:

Heaven's Jing Qi Shen nourishes and grows my Jin Dan...

Visualize your Jin Dan and body expanding from the size of Heaven to infinity, which is Tao. Chant:

Tao's Jing Qi Shen nourishes and grows my Jin Dan...

Now your Jin Dan and body stop rotating counterclockwise and start to rotate *clockwise*.
Visualize your Jin Dan reducing from the size of Tao to the size of Heaven.
Chant and visualize:

Tao and Tian Jing Qi Shen and Jing Hua (pronounced *dow, tyen jing chee shun, jing hwah*) *nourish and grow my true Jin Dan...*

Visualize your Jin Dan and body reducing from the size of Heaven to the size of Mother Earth.
Chant and visualize:

Tian and Di Jing Qi Shen and Jing Hua (pronounced *tyen, dee jing chee shun, jing hwah*) *nourish and grow my true Jin Dan...*

Visualize your Jin Dan and body reducing from the size of Mother Earth to the size of your body.
Chant and visualize:

Di and Body Jing Qi Shen and Jing Hua (pronounced *dee, jing chee shun, jing hwah*) *nourish and grow my true Jin Dan...*

Visualize your Jin Dan reducing from the size of your body to the size of the Ming Men acupuncture point.

Chant and visualize:

Tao Tian Di Ren Jing Qi Shen and Jing Hua He Yi (pronounced *dow tyen dee wren jing chee shun, jing hwah huh yee*) *nourish and grow my true Jin Dan*...

This Sacred Source Jin Dan Meditation will gather the jing qi shen from the body, Mother Earth, Heaven, and Tao to form and grow your Jin Dan. Jin Dan is one of the most sacred and powerful treasures for boosting energy, stamina, vitality, and immunity; for healing, rejuvenating, and prolonging life; and for transforming relationships, finances, and every aspect of life.

The Sacred Source Jin Dan Meditation is the sacred way to reach Tao. This is one of the most important spiritual practices for a human being. This is a daily practice. I am so grateful that I received this sacred meditation from The Source to share with humanity.

Tao is The Source that creates Heaven, Mother Earth, and countless planets, stars, galaxies, and universes. Heaven and Mother Earth are the creator of human beings.

Tao is The Way of all life.

Tao is the universal principles and laws.

A human being has two lives: physical life and soul life. A human being's physical life is limited. A human being's soul life is eternal. What is the ultimate goal of a human being's life? It can be summarized in one sentence:

The ultimate goal of a human being's life is to reach Tao.

This Sacred Source Jin Dan Meditation is a sacred Source practice to transform all life and reach Tao. The significance and power of this meditation cannot be expressed by words, comprehended by thoughts, or imagined.

Practice. Practice. Practice.
Boost energy, stamina, vitality, and immunity.
Heal soul, heart, mind, and body.
Prevent all sickness.

Purify soul, heart, mind, and body.
Rejuvenate soul, heart, mind, and body.
Enlighten soul, heart, mind, and body.
Prolong life.
Move in the direction of immortality.
Reach Tao.
Love you. Love you. Love you.
Thank you. Thank you. Thank you.

I am unbounded and free

I cannot thank Master Sha enough for the countless blessings I have received over the years. What we are receiving comes in many layers. I needed a lot of work, so I just decided to keep showing up over and over again. My greatest wish was always to live fully—natural, complete, and whole.

Over time the blessings have removed countless layers of blockages. This latest blessing for the Life Gate, the Ming Men, is truly incredible. I feel I have the power of the mountains, the rivers, the oceans, and the forests.

I am unbounded and free. I now move naturally in fulfillment of my true service and purpose. I now know I can complete my task. What greater blessing than to do what you love.

Thank you, Master Sha. Thank you, The Source.

Christopher Keehn
Monterey, California, U.S.A.

Back pain disappeared with Ming Men blessing

Beloved Master Sha,

Yesterday during your Sunday Divine Blessings teleconference I received the priceless treasure Ming Men Mi Zhou Soul Mind Body Transplants. The pain in my lower back that I had for several days instantly disappeared. Today I have so much energy and strength in both of my legs when walking.

Thank you for all the blessings we always receive during Sunday Divine Blessings. My heart is so full of gratitude and joy. With all my love to Master Sha, all layers of Heaven, and The Source.

Stanka
Tutzing, Germany

The Source Sacred Mantras
for Healing the Spiritual,
Mental, Emotional, and
Physical Bodies

THROUGHOUT HISTORY, chanting mantras has been one of the most important methods of spiritual and energy healing and development. Millions of healing stories have been created by chanting mantras.

In ancient teaching and practice, there are three secrets that I explained in chapter 1: Shen Mi (*Body Secret*), Kou Mi (*Mouth Secret*), and Yi Mi (*Thinking Secret*). Mouth Secret is to chant mantras. In 2000 I created the Four Power Techniques, which are Body Power, Soul Power, Mind Power, and Sound Power. Sound Power is to chant mantras.

In the books of my Soul Power Series and my other books, I have offered much teaching about many sacred mantras, ancient and new. I encourage you to read these books. I have shared many powerful mantras together with soul and ancient secrets, wisdom, knowledge, and practical techniques for applying mantras to self-heal and more. These teachings and practices have created hundreds of thousands of soul healing miracles worldwide.

I published two major books on healing before creating the Soul Power Series:

- *Power Healing: The Four Keys to Energizing Your Body, Mind, and Spirit*[15]
- *Soul Mind Body Medicine: A Complete Soul Healing System for Optimum Health and Vitality*[16]

My Soul Power Series consists so far of ten major books:[17]

- *Soul Wisdom: Practical Soul Treasures to Transform Your Life*
- *Soul Communication: Opening Your Spiritual Channels for Success and Fulfillment*
- *The Power of Soul: The Way to Heal, Rejuvenate, Transform, and Enlighten All Life*
- *Divine Soul Songs: Sacred Practical Treasures to Heal, Rejuvenate, and Transform You, Humanity, Mother Earth, and All Universes*
- *Divine Soul Mind Body Healing and Transmission System: The Divine Way to Heal You, Humanity, Mother Earth, and All Universes*
- *Tao I: The Way of All Life*
- *Divine Transformation: The Divine Way to Self-clear Karma to Transform Your Health, Relationships, Finances, and More*
- *Tao II: The Way of Healing, Rejuvenation, Longevity, and Immortality*
- *Tao Song and Tao Dance: Sacred Sound, Movement, and Power from The Source for Healing, Rejuvenation, Longevity, and Transformation of All Life*
- *Divine Healing Hands: Experience Divine Power to Heal You, Animals, and Nature, and to Transform All Life*

I have shared the most powerful mantras in history in these books. Billions of people throughout history have received transformation in every aspect of life through these sacred practices.

Let me emphasize again the power and significance of mantras.

---

[15] *Power Healing: The Four Keys to Energizing Your Body, Mind, and Spirit* (San Francisco: HarperSanFrancisco, 2002).

[16] *Soul Mind Body Medicine: A Complete Soul Healing System for Optimum Health and Vitality* (Novato: New World Library, 2006).

[17] See "Books of the Soul Power Series" section starting on page 277 for more information about each of these books.

What Is a Mantra?

A mantra is a special sound and message that the Divine, Tao, buddhas, saints, gurus, and other kinds of spiritual fathers and mothers created in their spiritual and energy practice for transforming all life. When a mantra is chanted repeatedly, transformation occurs.

The Power and Significance of Mantras

Mantras are special sounds and messages that carry high spiritual frequencies and vibrations. These special frequencies and vibrations can transform the frequency and vibration of all life.

Mantras carry love, forgiveness, compassion, and light. Love melts all blockages and transforms all life. Forgiveness brings inner joy and inner peace to all life. Compassion boosts energy, stamina, vitality, and immunity of all life. Light heals, prevents sickness, purifies and rejuvenates soul, heart, mind, and body, purifies and rejuvenates spiritual, mental, emotional, and physical bodies, transforms relationships and finances, increases intelligence, opens spiritual channels, and brings success in every aspect of all life.

Mantras are a spiritual gathering treasure. When you chant a mantra, the saints and spiritual fathers and mothers in Heaven hear you chanting and will come to bless your life.

Mantras are a major spiritual communication tool to communicate with the Soul World.

Chanting mantras is one of the most ancient spiritual practices. For thousands of years, renowned Hindu, Buddhist, Taoist, and other spiritual leaders in many different traditions have shared their mantras to serve millions of people.

Mantras are extremely powerful because they can remove soul mind body blockages in every aspect of life. I want to share and emphasize a major spiritual secret. When you chant a mantra, please do Forgiveness Practice at the same time. Forgiveness Practice is the key to self-clear negative karma. Negative karma is the root blockage in every aspect of life, including health, relationships, finances, business, and more. Remember, every time you chant a mantra, do Forgiveness Practice at the same time. It will enhance your healing and life transformation many times over. Let me explain further.

Negative karma is the record of one's mistakes in all lifetimes, including one's current lifetime and all past lifetimes. It also includes one's negative ancestral karma. Negative ancestral karma is the record of mistakes on your fathers' or mothers' ancestral side that affects your soul journey and your physical life as one of their descendants. Negative karma includes killing, harming, taking advantage of others, cheating, stealing, and causing others pain and suffering in any way.

Since July 2003 the Divine has given me the honor to offer Divine Karma Cleansing to humanity. Since February 2009 I have personally trained and created over thirty Divine Channels, who are also my Worldwide Representatives. They also offer Divine Karma Cleansing. Together we have offered Divine Karma Cleansing to hundreds of thousands of people on Mother Earth. In the last ten years we have created hundreds of thousands of soul healing miracles. We have also created more than four thousand Divine Healing Hands Soul Healers on Mother Earth. The teachings and practices of my Soul Power Series books, along with *Power Healing* and *Soul Mind Body Medicine*, have also created thousands of soul healing miracles.

How can we create so many soul healing miracles? Because we offer Divine Karma Cleansing and we teach self-healing. Most especially, we have taught Forgiveness Practice a lot. Forgiveness Practice is the sacred way to self-clear karma.

To self-clear karma is to ask for forgiveness for the mistakes that we and our ancestors have made in all lifetimes. Mistakes we have made created negative karma. Because of our negative karma, there is darkness with us. The darkness can stay inside us or around us. The darkness could be within our business or with our family members. Negative karma affects health, emotions, relationships, finances, business, home, family, and every aspect of life.

I revealed the one-sentence secret about karma in my book *The Power of Soul*:

**Karma is the root cause of success and failure
in every aspect of life.**

Our success depends on our good service in previous lives and this life. Our blockages are due to our unpleasant service in previous lives and this life. Our ancestors' karma also affects our life.

If you have received Divine Karma Cleansing, you are very blessed. If you have not received Divine Karma Cleansing, learn how to do Forgiveness Practice to self-clear your negative karma little by little. Even if you have received Divine Karma Cleansing, do Forgiveness Practice. In all of my books and in every workshop, seminar, and retreat I lead, I strongly emphasize the importance of Forgiveness Practice. I have personally witnessed the power of doing Forgiveness Practice. It is one of the golden keys to unlock the door to advancing in every aspect of life.

When you do Forgiveness Practice, not all of the darkness will leave right away. The darkness leaves little by little. Therefore, Forgiveness Practice is a daily practice.

When you do Forgiveness Practice, it is vital to include the following:

> *Dear all the darkness within my body,*
> *Please forgive me for all mistakes I have made in this lifetime and*
>   *any past lifetime to harm, hurt, or take advantage of you.*
> *I sincerely apologize.*
> *Please forgive me.*
>
> *Dear all souls and all people who have harmed, hurt, or taken*
>   *advantage of me in all lifetimes,*
> *I forgive all of you unconditionally.*

These are the two aspects of Forgiveness Practice:

- sincerely ask for forgiveness
- unconditionally forgive others

Asking the darkness to forgive you and offering unconditional forgiveness is the first key for the Forgiveness Practice. Now I will release the second key:

Ask the darkness inside your body to practice with you.

The sacred wisdom is that when you do spiritual practice, including chanting, meditating, and more, invite the darkness inside the body to practice with you. All beings need love, forgiveness, compassion, and light. The darkness needs love, forgiveness, compassion, and light also. Darkness also has a soul, mind, and body.

What are you doing when you are chanting and meditating? You are doing Xiu Lian. "Xiu Lian" (pronounced *sheo lyen*) means *purification practice*, and can be summarized in one sentence:

Xiu Lian is the purification practice of soul, heart, mind, and body in order to reach soul mind body enlightenment.

Xiu Lian represents the totality of the spiritual journey. You need Xiu Lian. The darkness that is the negative karma within you needs Xiu Lian also. To invite the darkness to chant and meditate with you is the absolute top secret for healing and transforming all life. Darkness is with you if your karma has not been cleared. Once your karma has been cleared, you do not need to invite the darkness to meditate with you. If your karma has not been cleared, you absolutely need to invite the darkness to meditate with you.

Do Forgiveness Practice every day. It is very difficult to self-clear all negative karma quickly. There could be high levels of negative karma. It takes time to clear negative karma. Therefore, Xiu Lian is not easy. In history many great spiritual masters went to the mountains, caves, temples, forests, and oceans to do Xiu Lian for decades. They wanted to clear their negative karma and enlighten their soul, mind, and body.

Therefore, when you meditate or chant, before you start always remember to say:

> *If there is darkness inside my body, please join me to chant and*
> *meditate.*
> *Let us do Xiu Lian together.*
> *Thank you.*

Remember, this is a major secret to self-clear negative karma.

Now I will share with you three powerful new The Source sacred mantras that I received directly from The Source. I am so honored.

Sacred Source Mantra *Tao Guang Zha Shan*

Tao is The Source. Tao is The Way of all life. Tao is the universal principles and laws. Tao carries Tao frequency and vibration with Tao jing qi shen that can transform the frequency, vibration, and jing qi shen of everyone and everything. Tao has the ultimate power for healing and transformation of all life. "Guang" (pronounced *gwahng*) means *light*. There is visible light and invisible light. "Zha" (pronounced *jah*) means *explodes*. "Shan" (pronounced *shahn*) means *vibrates*.

"Tao Guang Zha Shan" means *The Source light explodes and vibrates*.

All sickness is due to soul mind body blockages. The Source light has the power to remove soul mind body blockages. People who carry light negative karma could receive instant healing from The Source light. People who carry heavy negative karma could take more time to clear it. It does not matter if one receives instant healing or if it takes some time to heal; it still works.

I will emphasize again: **it is most important to do Forgiveness Practice with any soul healing practice.** That is the best way to remove soul mind body blockages in every aspect of life.

Now let us apply this new Source mantra for healing.

Heal the Physical Body

Remember Da Tao zhi jian, *The Big Way is extremely simple.* The soul healing and soul transformation techniques that I teach in this book and my previous books are extremely simple. They could be too simple to believe. Open your heart and soul to give them a try. Apply the techniques. *If you want to know if a pear is sweet, taste it. If you want to know if soul healing works, experience it.* If you experience instant results, you will believe soul healing works. If you do not experience instant results, be patient. Continue to practice. Transformation is on the way.

Why would a person not receive instant results? It would be because the person has heavy soul mind body blockages. For example, some people suffer with chronic pain for decades. It could take some time to completely heal. Some people suffer from life-threatening conditions. It takes time to heal. Most important is to follow my instructions. When I ask you to stop reading and practice for ten minutes, I cannot emphasize enough that you need to practice. That is the key for self-healing: *practice*. I want to remind you again of the message of soul healing miracles:

I have the power to create soul healing miracles
to transform all of my life.

You have the power to create soul healing miracles
to transform all of your life.

Together we have the power to create soul healing miracles
to transform all life of humanity and all souls in Mother Earth
and countless planets, stars, galaxies, and universes.

You *can* do it!

I also want to emphasize that for chronic or life-threatening conditions you need to practice two hours or more a day. You can add all of your practice time together to total at least two hours a day. Do the simple exercises I share in this book. Chant and visualize at the same time. Success can be yours if you practice.

The physical body includes every system, every organ, every cell, four extremities, and more. Sicknesses in the physical body include pain, inflammation, infection, cysts, stones, tumors, cancer, and much more. The cause of all sicknesses is soul mind body blockages. Soul blockages are negative karma. Mind blockages include negative mind-sets, negative attitudes, negative beliefs, ego, attachments, and more. Body blockages are energy and matter blockages. The Source mantra *Tao Guang Zha Shan* can remove all kinds of blockages. You could create soul healing miracles just by chanting this one mantra.

In the practices in the rest of this chapter, I will lead you to use Soul Power (Say Hello Healing and Blessing) to invoke three The Source Ling Guang ("Soul Light") Calligraphies—one for each of the three new Source sacred mantras I am introducing in this chapter. In chapter 5 I will offer much more teaching about The Source Ling Guang Calligraphies. I do not want you to wait to experience their power and receive their benefits.

Next I will give you a general formula for soul self-healing of all sickness in the physical body. This formula can be used for your entire life—anywhere, anytime. It is extremely simple.

Apply the Four Power Techniques and Forgiveness Practice together:

Body Power. Refer to the color insert near the end of chapter 5. Put one palm on figure 13, The Source Ling Guang Calligraphy *Tao Guang Zha Shan* (pronounced *dow gwahng jah shahn*). Put your other palm on any part of your body that needs healing.

Soul Power. Say *hello*.

Say *hello* to inner souls:

> *Dear soul mind body of* _____ (name any organ, system, or
>   part of your body that needs healing),
> *I love you.*
> *You have the power to heal yourself.*
> *Do a good job!*
> *Thank you.*

Say *hello* to outer souls and do Forgiveness Practice together:

> *Dear Divine,*
> *Dear Tao, The Source,*
> *Dear The Source Ling Guang Calligraphy* Tao Guang Zha Shan,
> *Dear countless healing angels, archangels, ascended masters, gurus,*
>   *lamas, kahunas, holy saints, Taoist saints, other saints, buddhas,*
>   *bodhisattvas, and all kinds of spiritual fathers and mothers who*
>   *are connected with The Source Ling Guang Calligraphy,*
> *Dear countless saints' animals who are connected with The Source*
>   *Ling Guang Calligraphy,*

Dear countless soul healing treasures that are connected with The
    Source Ling Guang Calligraphy,
I love you, honor you, and appreciate you.
Please forgive my ancestors and me for all of the mistakes that we
    have made in all lifetimes.
Please heal and rejuvenate my physical body.
I cannot honor you enough.
Thank you.

Dear all of the people and all the souls that my ancestors and I have
    hurt, harmed, or taken advantage of in the physical body in all
    lifetimes,
We sincerely apologize.
Please forgive my ancestors and me.
I am truly sorry.
Let us chant and meditate together to heal and rejuvenate our physical
    bodies.

Dear all souls who have hurt me in all lifetimes,
I forgive you unconditionally.
In order for me to be forgiven, I will offer unconditional service to
    humanity and all souls.
To chant Tao Guang Zha Shan *is to offer unconditional service.*
I am bringing Tao Guang to humanity and wan ling on Mother Earth
    and in countless planets, stars, galaxies, and universes.
Thank you.

Sound Power. Chant silently or aloud:

Tao Guang Zha Shan (pronounced *dow gwahng jah shahn*)
Tao Guang Zha Shan
Tao Guang Zha Shan
Tao Guang Zha Shan
Tao Guang Zha Shan
Tao Guang Zha Shan
Tao Guang Zha Shan . . .

The Source light explodes and vibrates.
The Source light explodes and vibrates.
The Source light explodes and vibrates.
The Source light explodes and vibrates.
The Source light explodes and vibrates.
The Source light explodes and vibrates.
The Source light explodes and vibrates…

Mind Power. Visualize Tao Guang (*Source light*) exploding and vibrating in the area of your request.

Keep your hands in the same position: one hand on the area of your request, the other on figure 13. Chant and visualize for ten minutes.

At the end of every healing practice, always remember to show your gratitude:

Hao! Hao! Hao!
Thank you. Thank you. Thank you.
Gong Song. Gong Song. Gong Song.

"Gong Song" (pronounced *gohng sohng*) is Chinese for *respectfully return*. This is to return the countless souls who came for the Forgiveness Practice.

"Hao" (pronounced *how*) means *get well*. "Hao" means *perfect*. "Hao" means *restore health*.

For chronic or life-threatening conditions, practice for a half-hour or more each time and practice several times every day. Your daily practice time *must* total at least two hours. This is Heaven's Guidance that I have consistently received for more than ten years: for chronic or life-threatening conditions, *practice at least two hours every day*.

You can use the same approach to heal your spiritual body, mental body, and emotional body. The techniques will be the same, but your specific healing requests will differ.

Miracle mantra heals severe leg pain

Chanting the mantra Tao Guang Zha Shan is a practice that everyone should do.

I wake up almost every day with pain in my legs, especially my knees, ankles, and feet. My pain on a scale of 1 to 10 is usually 7 or higher, and at night or in the afternoon it's 8 to 9. Sometimes when I get up from a seated position I can hardly stand. It's like my legs are heavy and painful.

In the daily Free Divine Healing Hands Blessings teleconference we practiced this mantra for over forty minutes. I asked the soul of this sacred mantra to heal my legs. I was cleaning my house after that and realized that the pain reduced from 8 to 2—almost gone! My legs feel strong, youthful, and pain-free. You need to experience this healing power. If I want to improve my condition, the answer is very easy: I need to chant more.

Tao Guang Zha Shan, Tao Guang Zha Shan, Tao Guang Zha Shan, Tao Guang Zha Shan...

I'm going to start practicing this mantra every day for me and my loved ones.

Thank you, Master Sha, for sharing your love and service with us and for teaching us this sacred miracle mantra. There are no words to express my gratitude, my happiness to be pain-free, and my love. Thank you!

Carmelita
Tucson, Arizona, U.S.A.

Sadness totally relieved by *Tao Guang Zha Shan* mantra

I experienced the great power of the new mantra of The Source, Tao Guang Zha Shan. I never experienced anything so powerful before. For the past two weeks I have been in spiritual testing: so sad and without energy or motivation to do anything.

During the Sunday Divine Blessings teleconference, I was sleeping near my computer for a few hours and suddenly woke up during your chanting of this mantra that I had never heard before. I felt that this was very powerful. Instantly, my energy came back. I felt peace and joy in my heart. I felt more grounded, and it is ongoing. I cannot stop chanting this mantra; I love it so much.

I feel every day the power that is transforming my life now, removing mind blockages such as ego of inferiority that I see clearly. I wake up lighter and with joy and trust in my heart.

May this wonderful and powerful mantra help as many people as possible who suffer from sadness, depression, and lack of energy. I cannot thank you enough, Master Sha, for bringing this light and transformation to humanity. I cannot thank the Divine and The Source enough for helping us all to heal and remove our blockages. I am very grateful.

M. L.
Canada

Sciatica pain greatly reduced by two minutes of chanting

During the Sunday Divine Blessings teleconference, Master Sha offered a blessing by chanting the Tao Guang Zha Shan *mantra for two minutes. I asked for my sciatic nerve to be healed. I've suffered with sciatica in my right hip area all the way down the leg for thirty-five years after a car accident. I felt heat all over, and after two minutes of chanting with Master Sha, the intense pain was greatly reduced. I slept that night without the intense pain for the first time.*

C. S.
Tampa, Florida, U.S.A.

Heaven comes to Mother Earth with every word

The practice with the new mantras Tao Guang Zha Shan, Hei Heng Hong Ha, Guang Liang Hao Mei *brought such high frequencies and light to Mother Earth and to each person. When stomping on the ground and chanting the mantras together as a group, I felt a very strong connection between The Source and Mother Earth, and received a particularly good grounding.*

Heaven comes to Mother Earth with every word of these mantras—so much radiant, powerful, and bright light that did not exist before.

I received blessings for my legs. For the last year I have suffered often with a lot of pain and little power in my legs, making it very hard for me to run. Now I feel a much better connection to Mother Earth and can feel roots that extend into the interior of the earth. It vibrates comfortably in my legs. The connection to The Source is much more intense and I feel balance within me.

Thank you, dear Master Sha, for these wonderful healing mantras. I cannot thank you enough.

Birgit Seefeldt
Bad Freienwalde, Germany

Love, light, and healing on every layer of my being

Aloha Master Sha,

I am very excited for each new day as I grow and learn with you.

The new mantra Tao Guang Zha Shan *is so powerful in my body that all my energy centers, systems, my brain, my soul, and my spiritual team LOVE this new mantra, and the feelings and images that I have been receiving are very profound!*

I feel great, strong, healed, loved, and supported. Most of all, I am healed! On every layer of my being there is light, love, and healing taking place.

Thank you for your service to us ALL.

With light and love to you!

Dove S.

Sacred Source Mantra *Hei Heng Hong Ha*

Now let us learn, practice, and experience the second new Source mantra and the second Source Ling Guang Calligraphy in this book.

"Hei" (pronounced *hay*) is the sacred sound that stimulates the first (root) energy chakra, which is the first Soul House. Millions of people understand the energy chakras. See figure 9 on page 56 to understand where they are located. The Divine and Tao asked me to emphasize that the energy chakras are the *Soul Houses*. Our beloved body soul resides in one of the seven energy chakras. Therefore, in my teaching, the energy chakras are called the Soul Houses.

"Heng" (pronounced *hung*) is the sacred sound that stimulates the second energy chakra or second Soul House.

"Hong" (pronounced *hawng*) is the sacred sound that stimulates the third energy chakra or third Soul House.

"Ha" (pronounced *hah*) is the sacred sound to stimulate the Zhong.

Hei Heng Hong Ha are the four sacred sounds to stimulate the first, second, and third Soul Houses, as well as the Zhong. See figure 14.

I introduced the Zhong briefly near the end of chapter 1. "Zhong" means *core*. The Zhong (pronounced *jawng*) is an area in the back half of the lower abdomen that includes four major sacred areas and points. They are the Hui Yin acupuncture point, Kun Gong, Ming Men acupuncture point, and Wei Lü. See figure 12 on page 63.

The Hui Yin (pronounced *hway yeen*) acupuncture point lies on the perineum, between the genitals and the anus. "Hui" means *accumulation*. "Yin" means *yin energy*. The Hui Yin point gathers the yin energy of one's whole body.

The Kun Gong is located in the center of the body behind the navel. As explained in the sacred Immortal Tao Jing,[18] the Kun Gong is located above and in front of the kidneys, below the heart, to the left of the liver, and to the right of the spleen.

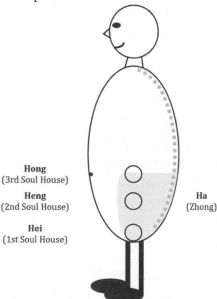

Hong
(3rd Soul House)

Heng
(2nd Soul House)

Hei
(1st Soul House)

Ha
(Zhong)

FIGURE 14. Hei Heng Hong Ha stimulates the body

---

[18] The Immortal Tao Jing or Immortal Tao Classic is a new 220-line sacred text from Tao. It is the principal subject of my book *Tao II: The Way of Healing, Rejuvenation, Longevity, and Immortality* (Toronto/New York: Heaven's Library/Atria Books, 2010).

In the *I Ching*, "Kun" means *Mother Earth* or *Mother's energy*. "Gong" means *temple*. Kun Gong (pronounced *kwun gawng*) is the sacred place to produce Yuan Qi and Yuan Jing. "Yuan" means *origin*. "Yuan Qi" (pronounced *ywen chee*) means *original energy*. "Yuan Jing" (pronounced *ywen jing*) means *original matter*. Yuan Qi and Yuan Jing are the keys for life. Yuan Jing and Yuan Qi are produced in the Kun Gong.

Yuan Qi, Yuan Jing, and Yuan Shen are the true life force for a human being. Yuan Shen is the original soul. The sacred wisdom is when the father's sperm and mother's egg join together to create an embryo, Tao (The Source) gives Yuan Shen to this embryo. Yuan Shen creates Yuan Qi (original energy) and Yuan Jing (original matter). Think of an oil lamp. Yuan Shen, Yuan Qi, and Yuan Jing are just like the oil in a lamp. The jing qi shen of the whole body is also oil in the lamp. At birth, a healthy baby has a full bottle of oil. Yuan Qi and Yuan Jing are fulfilled. Sickness, aging, and other factors deplete one's oil. Yuan Qi and Yuan Jing are depleted. This is the normal process for a human being. When one's oil is completely exhausted, physical life ends. Therefore, Yuan Shen, Yuan Qi, and Yuan Jing are the true life force for a human being.

Kun Gong is the place to produce Yuan Qi and Yuan Jing. No physical exercise, special food, liquids, or nutrients can replenish Yuan Qi and Yuan Jing. Normal spiritual practice cannot replenish this true life force either. Only sacred spiritual practices can develop Yuan Qi and Yuan Jing. To develop Yuan Qi and Yuan Jing is to replenish the bottle of life oil.

This is one of the most important teachings that the Divine and Tao gave to me to share with humanity. This is one of the most important secrets that I offer in my ten-year longevity and immortality training. If you are truly inspired and desire to learn sacred wisdom, knowledge, and practical techniques of rejuvenation and longevity, please read my books *Tao I: The Way of All Life, Tao II: The Way of Healing, Rejuvenation, Longevity, and Immortality,* and *Tao Song and Tao Dance: Sacred Sound, Movement, and Power from The Source for Healing, Rejuvenation, Longevity, and Transformation of All Life.*[19] You can also join my Tao Healing, Rejuvenation, and Longevity Retreats.

---

[19] Toronto/New York: Heaven's Library/Atria Books, 2010-2012

The Ming Men acupuncture point lies on the back, directly behind the navel. (See figure 8 on page 54.) I offered teachings on the power and significance of the Ming Men acupuncture point in chapter 3. See pages 111–129.

The Wei Lü (pronounced *way lü*) is the tailbone area. (See figure 12 on page 63.) It is a sacred area where qi is generated and gathers. It is also a portal to an invisible hole in the bottom of the spinal column. This invisible hole is a gate for energy and tiny matter to enter and travel along the spinal column and the spinal cord.

Two major books in my Soul Power Series, *Divine Soul Songs* and *Tao Song and Tao Dance*, explain the seven Soul Houses in detail. I won't repeat the details, but I will give the essence for those of you who have not read these two books. If you have already read these two books, learn and master the essence.

The **first Soul House** is located just above the perineum, which is the area between the genitals and anus. It is fist-sized and located in the central channel of the body. The power and significance of the first Soul House can be summarized as follows:

- It is the foundation energy center for the other energy chakras or Soul Houses.
- It gathers the yin of the whole body.
- It is the key area to clear relationship karma.
- It is the key Soul House or energy chakra for healing and rejuvenation of the reproductive system and immune system; for healing the anus, rectum, and sexual organs; and for increasing sexual power.
- It is the sacred powerhouse for developing confidence and stability.
- It is the sacred powerhouse for longevity.
- It is the sacred powerhouse for singing Tao Song or Soul Song.

The **second Soul House** is located in the central channel of the body in the lower abdomen, between the first Soul House and the level of the navel. It is also fist-sized. The power and significance of the second Soul House can be summarized as follows:

- It is the key Soul House for empowering the Lower Dan Tian, which is one of the most important foundation energy centers in the body. The Lower Dan Tian is located 1.5 cun[20] below the navel and 2.5 cun inside the front of the body, and is fist-sized.
- It is the sacred powerhouse for rejuvenation.
- It is a key Soul House for boosting energy, stamina, vitality, and immunity.
- It is a key Soul House for healing the large intestine.
- It is a sacred powerhouse for losing weight.

The **third Soul House** is located in the central channel of the body at the level of the navel. It is also fist-sized. The power and significance of the third Soul House can be summarized as follows:

- It is the key Soul House for empowering, healing, and rejuvenating the Water element, which includes the kidneys, urinary bladder, ears, and bones in the physical body and fear in the emotional body.
- It is the key Soul House for empowering, healing, and rejuvenating the Wood element, which includes the liver, gallbladder, eyes, and tendons in the physical body and anger in the emotional body.
  - It is the key Soul House for healing and rejuvenating the urinary system and musculoskeletal system.
  - It is the key Soul House for healing and rejuvenating the stomach and small intestine.
  - It is key for empowering and developing the Snow Mountain Area and the Ming Men acupuncture point, which is located on the back, directly behind the navel.
- The Snow Mountain Area is the foundation energy center at the base of the spine and in front of the tailbone. It is known to yogis as kundalini, to Taoists as the Golden Urn, and to traditional Chinese medicine practitioners as the Ming Men area, which means *gate of life*.

---

[20] One cun (pronounced *tsoon*) equals the width of the thumb joint.

- The greatest power and significance of the Ming Men acupuncture point is that it is the Tao point for a human being, as I explained in chapter 3.
- The Snow Mountain Area and Ming Men acupuncture point carry Ming Men fire and Ming Men water. The Ming Men acupuncture point is the core of the Snow Mountain Area. Ming Men fire is the most important yang for the whole body. Ming Men water is the most important yin for the whole body. Millions of people suffer from hypertension, diabetes, or menopausal issues. From the perspective of energy, matter, and traditional Chinese medicine, all three of these unhealthy conditions are due to an insufficiency of Ming Men water. Sacred Source mantras have the power to heal these three unhealthy conditions and much, much more.
- The third Soul House supplies energy food for the brain and Third Eye through the Snow Mountain area.
- It is the key sacred powerhouse for developing courage, strength, fortitude, and persistence to overcome challenges.
- It is the key sacred powerhouse for developing jing, which is matter.

The **Zhong** is the Tao area in the body, located in the back half of the lower abdomen. The Ming Men acupuncture point is *the essence of the Zhong*. The power and significance of the Zhong can be summarized as follows:

- It is the core of life.
- It includes four major sacred areas and points: Kun Gong, Ming Men acupuncture point, Wei Lü, and Hui Yin acupuncture point.
- It is the most important sacred center for boosting energy, stamina, vitality, and immunity.
- It is the key center for rejuvenation and prolonging life.
- It is the sacred center for healing all sickness in the spiritual, mental, emotional, and physical bodies.
- It is the sacred center to transform all life, including relationships and finances.
- It is the sacred center for increasing intelligence.

Infused with heavenly energy

Today on the Free Divine Healing Hands Blessings teleconference we chanted The Source Soul Healing Mantra Hei Heng Hong Ha. Together with Master Lynne, we turned on our Divine Healing Hands and all our treasures. We began to chant silently. An exquisite feeling came over me and entered through the top of my head. It was as though I was being infused with the energy of a heavenly city. My heart opened.

After chanting for about fifteen minutes, I felt a sharp pain in my Ming Men area. I saw dark energy rise up my spinal cord and leave through the top of my head. Simultaneously, as I was focusing into my Zhong area, my consciousness expanded. I became aware of energy circles moving through my body and in my Third Eye there came a beautiful light. As I watched this light, I felt that I connected to the joy of my soul. The light formed pyramids and spun like a whirling vortex.

Our family cat, Mara, came and lay down beside me. She and I and Master Lynne and all the people on the teleconference line became one. I was happy and peaceful. Thank you, Master Sha and The Source, for this most beautiful gift. Every day you give us so much. I am so very grateful.

All my love,

Kathleen M.
Pennsylvania, U.S.A.

Let us now do a practice with *Hei Heng Hong Ha* and The Source Ling Guang Calligraphy *Hei Heng Hong Ha*. This Source mantra could heal all sickness and transform all life. I will lead you to do a practice for healing the emotional body.

Heal the Emotional Body

Five thousand years ago, traditional Chinese medicine clearly shared the connection between the physical body and the emotional body. The physical body and emotional body are connected through the Five Elements.

Anger in the emotional body connects with the Wood element. The authority organ of the Wood element is the liver. Anger is the emotional body; the liver is the physical body. They are interrelated. Anger could cause liver sickness. Liver sickness could cause anger. To heal anger is to heal the liver. To heal the liver is to heal anger.

In the same way, depression and anxiety in the emotional body connect with the Fire element. The authority organ of the Fire element is the heart. To heal the heart is to heal depression and anxiety and vice versa.

Worry in the emotional body connects with the Earth element. The spleen is the authority organ of the Earth element. To heal the spleen is to heal worry and vice versa.

Grief and sadness in the emotional body connect with the Metal element. The lungs are the authority organ of the Metal element. To heal the lungs is to heal grief and sadness and vice versa.

Fear in the emotional body connects with the Water element. The kidneys are the authority organ of the Water element. To heal the kidneys is to heal fear and vice versa.

Now I will lead you to apply the Four Power Techniques for healing the emotional body:

Body Power. Sit up straight. Refer to the color insert near the end of chapter 5. Put one palm on figure 15, The Source Ling Guang Calligraphy *Hei Heng Hong Ha*. Put the other palm over the organ that is related to the emotional imbalance you wish to heal.

I will now share the relationships between the physical zang organs and the unbalanced emotions through the Five Elements in greater detail:

- Wood: Liver—anger, irritation, frustration, annoyance, rage, fury, resentment

- Fire: Heart—depression, anxiety, nervousness, self-love issues, guilt, misery, unhappiness, melancholy, gloominess
- Earth: Spleen—worry, concern, apprehension, burden
- Metal: Lungs—grief, sadness, sorrow, heartache, anguish, angst, pain, unhappiness, woe
- Water: Kidneys—fear, fright, terror, panic, distress, trepidation

For example, if you have any issues of depression, anxiety, nervousness, self-love, guilt, misery, unhappiness, melancholy, or gloominess, this is the way to practice:

Body Power. Put one palm on figure 15, The Source Ling Guang Calligraphy *Hei Heng Hong Ha*. Put your other palm over your heart.

Soul Power. Say *hello*:

Say *hello* to inner souls:

> *Dear soul mind body of my heart,*
> *I love you.*
> *You have the power to heal my* _____ (name the emotional
>   imbalance).
> *Do a good job!*
> *Thank you.*

Say *hello* to outer souls and do Forgiveness Practice together:

> *Dear Divine*
> *Dear Tao, The Source,*
> *Dear The Source Ling Guang Calligraphy* Hei Heng Hong Ha,
> *Dear countless healing angels, archangels, ascended masters, gurus,*
>   *lamas, kahunas, holy saints, Taoist saints, other saints, buddhas,*
>   *bodhisattvas, and all kinds of spiritual fathers and mothers who are*
>   *connected with The Source Ling Guang Calligraphy* Hei Heng Hong
>   Ha,

Dear countless saints' animals who are connected with The Source
   Ling Guang Calligraphy Hei Heng Hong Ha,
Dear countless soul healing treasures that are connected with The
   Source Ling Guang Calligraphy Hei Heng Hong Ha,
I love you, honor you, and appreciate you.
Please forgive my ancestors and me for all of the mistakes that we
   have made in all lifetimes.
Please heal my _____ (name the emotional imbalance).
I cannot honor you enough.
Thank you.

Dear all the people and all the souls who my ancestors and I have
   harmed, hurt, and taken advantage of in the emotional body in all
   lifetimes,
We sincerely apologize.
Please forgive my ancestors and me unconditionally.
Let us chant and meditate together to transform our emotional
   bodies.

Dear all souls who have harmed, hurt, and taken advantage of me in
   this lifetime and past lifetimes, I forgive you unconditionally.
In order for me to be forgiven, I will offer unconditional service to
   humanity and all souls.
To chant Hei Heng Hong Ha *is to offer unconditional service.*
I am bringing Hei Heng Hong Ha *to humanity and wan ling on*
   Mother Earth and in countless planets, stars, galaxies, and
   universes.

Sound Power. Chant silently or aloud:

Hei Heng Hong Ha (pronounced *hay hung hawng hah*)
Hei Heng Hong Ha
Hei Heng Hong Ha
Hei Heng Hong Ha
Hei Heng Hong Ha
Hei Heng Hong Ha

Hei Heng Hong Ha…

Mind Power. Visualize golden light of The Source radiating and vibrating in and around your heart.

Stop reading now. Meditate, visualize, and chant *Hei Heng Hong Ha* for ten minutes.

Close the practice: *Hao! Hao! Hao! Thank you. Thank you. Thank you. Gong Song. Gong Song. Gong Song.* Pronounced *gohng sohng*, this is Chinese for *respectfully return*. This is to return the countless souls who came for the Forgiveness Practice.

If you have a chronic or life-threatening condition, chant for two hours or more per day. The more often you chant and the longer you chant, the better the results you could receive. Add all of your practice time together to total at least two hours per day.

No medication needed

Since my childhood, for about twenty years now, I have suffered from severe hay fever. When it is at its worst during the summer, I have reactions in my skin, digestive system, nose, lungs, and eyes. My overall well-being is very reduced. I have pain all over my body and no energy. During this time I do have to take medication to control these symptoms, but they are only partially alleviated.

During a recent daily Free Divine Healing Hands Blessings teleconference, Master Sha introduced the new mantras Tao Guang Zha Shan, Hei Heng Hong Ha, *and* Guang Liang Hao Mei. *I wrote these sacred mantras down to memorize them and took the paper with me to work. There I did a "Say Hello" greeting and chanted these mantras. That evening I realized I had forgotten to take the medicine, and I was truly shocked to observe that I didn't have any hay fever symptoms at all!*

Today was my third straight day without medication, and still no symptoms! I can't remember even two days during summertime without medication and without any kind of symptoms! I am truly astounded by the healing power of these new mantras. Just a few minutes of chanting, and no more symptoms!

I am so extremely grateful. I cannot thank Master Sha, the Divine, The Source, and the sacred mantras enough for this soul healing miracle! May as many people as possible learn these mantras and practice with them to experience their soul healing miracles!

N. K.
Germany

Vision improves after minutes of chanting Source mantras
Dear Master Sha,

   The new The Source healing mantras are extremely powerful and a huge service and gift for humanity. My whole body is filled with light and energy.

   As we chanted, I asked for a blessing for my eyes, and only a few minutes of chanting made a great difference. My vision is clearer and my eyes are much more relaxed.

   We are very honored and blessed. Thank you.

E. K.
Frankfurt, Germany

   Now I will guide you to learn and practice the third new Source mantra I am releasing in this book, and also receive blessings from The Source Ling Guang Calligraphy for this mantra.

Sacred Source Mantra *Guang Liang Hao Mei*

"Guang" (pronounced *gwahng*) means *light*. This light includes the light of Mother Earth, the light of Heaven, and the light of Tao, The Source. "Liang" (pronounced *lyahng*) means *transparency*. Transparency is also light. This light can go through the organs and the body. In one's spiritual journey the highest achievement is to transform the physical body to a light body. This is Body Enlightenment. When your body has become a light body, a person with advanced Third Eye abilities can see through your body as though it were transparent. Transparency is very important for healing and to uplift one's soul journey.

   The new Source mantra "Guang Liang Hao Mei" (pronounced *gwahng lyahng how may*) means *transparent light brings inner and outer beauty.*

Layers of a Human Body

I am sharing another major spiritual secret. A human being's body has two layers. One layer is named *You Xing*. "You Xing" (pronounced *yoe shing*) means *has shape and can be seen*. The other layer is named *Wu Xing*. "Wu Xing" (pronounced *woo shing*) means *has no shape and cannot be seen*.

You Xing further divides into three sub-layers. Wu Xing also further divides into three sub-layers.

Put them together and the six layers of a human being's body are as follows:

You Xing

The sub-layers of You Xing are:

- capillary system
- organs
- systems

Wu Xing

The sub-layers of Wu Xing are:

- meridian system
- transparency
- light

I am delighted to share with each of you that we are directly working at the highest layers. The highest layers are light and transparency. Therefore, when we chant *Guang Liang*, which is "light" and "transparency," and visualize an area of our body shining the brightest light and becoming transparent, it is the highest spiritual and energy healing we can do.

We are extremely blessed that The Source has released this wisdom and practice. I am extremely honored to be a servant of the Divine, Tao, The Source, and humanity.

"Hao" (pronounced *how*), the third word of this new Source mantra, means *get well*. "Hao" means *perfect*. "Hao" means *restore your health to the normal condition.* When we do healing, we need to restore health to the normal condition. We need good health.

"Mei" (pronounced *may*), the fourth and final word of this new Source mantra, means *beauty*. In my teaching, there is inner beauty and outer beauty. Inner beauty is qualities of the soul, mind, and body. Outer beauty is also qualities of the soul, mind and body. "Mei" includes inner beauty and outer beauty.

Inner Beauty of the Soul

Inner beauty of the soul includes:

- love
- forgiveness
- compassion
- light
- kindness
- generosity
- sincerity
- honesty
- integrity
- humility
- purity
- grace
- selflessness
- virtue
- total GOLD[21] (to the Divine, Tao, and The Source)
- and much more

Inner Beauty of the Mind

Inner beauty of the mind includes:

- peace
- calmness

---

[21] Total GOLD is an acronym. G denotes *gratitude*. O denotes *obedience*. L denotes *loyalty*. D denotes *devotion*. Total GOLD to the Divine, Tao, The Source, and all of Heaven is a key to the spiritual journey.

- gratitude
- joy
- bliss
- acceptance
- selflessness
- positivity
- harmony
- clarity
- purity
- confidence
- flexibility
- creativity
- inspiration
- non-attachment
- and more

Inner Beauty of the Body

Inner beauty of the body includes:

- health
- energy
- strength
- flexibility
- flow
- balance
- purity
- harmony
- freedom
- attunement
- and more

Outer Beauty of the Soul, Mind, and Body

Outer beauty of the soul, mind, and body includes:

- actions radiating love, forgiveness, compassion, and light

- behaviors carrying sincerity, integrity, kindness, gentleness, and warmth
- speech overflowing with love, care, compassion, and light, and resonating with inspiration that is heart-touching and moving
- thoughts offering grace, care, humility, purity, gratitude, and service
- a body vibrating with health, fitness, groundedness, openness, and appeal
- and more

The sacred wisdom is that inner beauty brings outer beauty. It is important for people to realize this wisdom.

Meditation and chanting are spiritual practices that directly enhance and bring out one's inner beauty. At the same time, they develop and bring out one's outer beauty. You may know of spiritual beings who are radiantly beautiful. They radiate divine love and light and other divine qualities. To have great inner and outer beauty is one of the greatest benefits that everyone can achieve through meditation and chanting.

Soul Orders

My book *The Power of Soul: The Way to Heal, Rejuvenate, Transform, and Enlighten All Life*[22] includes an entire chapter about Soul Orders. Soul Orders are sacred wisdom and practice.

What is a Soul Order? An emperor or a president of a country can give an order. In the military, a general can give an order. In a company, a chief officer or owner can give an order. In a family, parents can give an order to their children. A judge can give an order. To send an order is to command action.

Soul Orders are sacred treasures for healing and prevention of sickness; rejuvenation of soul, heart, mind, and body; and transformation of relationships, finances, business, and every aspect of life.

Everything is made of soul, mind, and body. Soul, mind, and body are shen qi jing. *Soul is the boss.* When the soul gives an order, the mind and body will act to accomplish the order. When your soul gives an order, your mind and body will follow. This is the power of soul.

---

[22] Toronto/New York: Heaven's Library/Atria Books, 2009.

This is *soul over matter*. This is soul healing, soul rejuvenation, and soul transformation.

"Hao" is a Soul Order. When people are sick, it does not matter whether the sickness is at the level of the spiritual, mental, emotional, or physical body. The goal of soul healing and any healing modality is to restore health in order to get well. "Hao" means *get well*. "Hao" means *restore health*. Therefore, "Hao" is a Soul Order. It is so simple yet so powerful that it is beyond comprehension.

"Mei" (*beauty,* pronounced *may*) includes inner beauty and outer beauty. "Mei" is a Soul Order also.

"Guang Liang Hao Mei" (pronounced *gwahng lyahng how may*) is a Soul Order. "Guang Liang Hao Mei" means *transparent light brings inner and outer beauty*.

There are countless mantras in all kinds of spiritual practices and traditions. Why are mantras so powerful? In one sentence:

Mantras are Soul Orders.

The sacred wisdom of mantras is *what you chant is what you become*.

Now let us practice this third new sacred Source mantra together with The Source Ling Guang Calligraphy of this mantra to heal the mental body and spiritual body.

"Mind" means *consciousness*. There are many kinds of mind blockages, including negative mind-sets, negative beliefs, negative attitudes, ego, attachments, and more. Mental confusion, mental disorders, poor memory, difficulty concentrating, and lack of focus are several other common blockages of the mind.

There are also many kinds of spiritual blockages. Spiritual blockages (soul blockages) are negative karma. I will emphasize again: negative karma is the record of mistakes that one and one's ancestors have made in all lifetimes. They include killing, harming, taking advantage of others, lying, cheating, stealing, and much more.

Forgiveness Practice plus The Source mantra *Guang Liang Hao Mei* are priceless treasures to heal the mental body and spiritual body. Of course, this sacred Source mantra can also heal the emotional body and physical body.

As an example, I will lead you in a practice using these treasures to heal the mental body and spiritual body.

Apply the Four Power Techniques:

Body Power. Refer to the color insert near the end of chapter 5. Put one palm on figure 16, The Source Ling Guang Calligraphy *Guang Liang Hao Mei*. Put your other palm over your heart. Traditional Chinese medicine teaches that the heart houses the mind and soul. Just as the body soul is the boss of the mind and body, the soul of the heart is the soul leader for the souls of all systems, organs, and cells.

Soul Power. Say *hello*:

Say *hello* to inner souls:

> *Dear soul mind body of my heart and mind,*
> *I love you both.*
> *You have the power to heal my _____ (name your spiritual and mental challenges).*
> *Do a good job!*
> *Thank you.*

Say *hello* to outer souls and do Forgiveness Practice together:

> *Dear Divine,*
> *Dear Tao, The Source,*
> *Dear The Source Ling Guang Calligraphy Guang Liang Hao Mei,*
> *Dear countless healing angels, archangels, ascended masters, gurus, lamas, kahunas, holy saints, Taoist saints, other saints, buddhas, bodhisattvas, and all kinds of spiritual fathers and mothers who are connected with The Source Ling Guang Calligraphy Guang Liang Hao Mei,*
> *Dear countless saints' animals who are connected with The Source Ling Guang Calligraphy Guang Liang Hao Mei,*
> *Dear countless soul healing treasures that are connected with The Source Ling Guang Calligraphy Guang Liang Hao Mei,*

I love you, honor you, and appreciate you.
Please forgive my ancestors and me for all of the mistakes that we
*   have made in all lifetimes.*
Please heal my _____ (name your spiritual and mental
*   challenges).*
I cannot honor you enough.
Thank you.

Dear all of the people and all the souls that my ancestors and I have
*   harmed, hurt, or taken advantage of in the mental and spiritual*
*   bodies in all lifetimes,*
We sincerely apologize.
Please forgive my ancestors and me unconditionally.
Let us chant and meditate together to transform our mental and
*   spiritual bodies.*
Dear all souls who have harmed, hurt, or taken advantage of me in
*   all my lifetimes in my mental or spiritual bodies, I forgive you*
*   unconditionally.*
In order to be forgiven, I will offer unconditional service to humanity
*   and all souls.*
To chant Guang Liang Hao Mei *is to offer unconditional service.*
I am bringing Guang Liang Hao Mei *to humanity and wan ling*
*   on Mother Earth and in countless planets, stars, galaxies, and*
*   universes.*

Sound Power. Chant silently or aloud:

Guang Liang Hao Mei (pronounced *gwahng lyahng how may*)
Guang Liang Hao Mei
Guang Liang Hao Mei
Guang Liang Hao Mei
Guang Liang Hao Mei
Guang Liang Hao Mei
Guang Liang Hao Mei…

Light, transparency, get well, inner and outer beauty

Light, transparency, get well, inner and outer beauty
Light, transparency, get well, inner and outer beauty
Light, transparency, get well, inner and outer beauty
Light, transparency, get well, inner and outer beauty
Light, transparency, get well, inner and outer beauty
Light, transparency, get well, inner and outer beauty . . .

Mind Power. Visualize rainbow light from The Source radiating in and around your heart and mind.

Stop reading. Continue to keep one hand on the calligraphy and one hand over the heart. Continue to chant *Guang Liang Hao Mei* and *light, transparency, get well, inner and outer beauty* for ten minutes.

Close the practice: *Hao! Hao! Hao! Thank you. Thank you. Thank you. Gong Song. Gong Song. Gong Song.* Pronounced *gohng sohng*, this is Chinese for *respectfully return*. This is to return the countless souls who came for the Forgiveness Practice.

You can use the same practice to heal the physical body and emotional body. Apply the Four Power Techniques and make the appropriate changes to the Soul Power and more.

I will emphasize again: in order to create your own soul healing miracles, do not skip the ten minutes of practice. For chronic or life-threatening conditions, practice much longer. Add all of your practice times together to total at least two hours a day. In the last ten years, the Four Power Techniques and soul healing have created hundreds of thousands of soul healing miracles. Therefore, the Divine and Tao guided me to write this new Soul Healing Miracles series.

The power and significance of the new Source mantras, *Tao Guang Zha Shan* (The Source light explodes and vibrates), *Hei Heng Hong Ha* (The Source Special Mantra for Zhong), and *Guang Liang Hao Mei* (light, transparency, get well, inner and outer beauty), can be summarized as follows:

- These mantras carry The Source frequency and vibration with Source love, forgiveness, compassion, and light that could remove soul mind body blockages of sickness to heal the spiritual, mental, emotional, and physical bodies.
- These mantras carry The Source field of Source jing qi shen that can transform the jing qi shen of the spiritual, mental, emotional, and physical bodies.
- These mantras carry the power of The Source to empower everyone to boost energy, stamina, vitality, and immunity.
- These mantras carry The Source abilities to transform all life, including transforming relationships, finances, business, intelligence, and every aspect of life.

The Soul Light Era started on August 8, 2003. It will last fifteen thousand years. It is now August 2013. The Soul Light Era is only ten years old. The three new Source mantras can serve billions of people in the Soul Light Era by empowering them to create their own soul healing miracles to transform all life.

We are extremely honored.

We are extremely blessed.

Much more clarity and light

This evening's meditation in front of The Source Ling Guang Calligraphy was deeply relaxing. The meditation was extremely powerful. I felt like I might take off like a rocket ship, there was so much energy and vibration moving through my feet.

My Message Center expanded out in all directions. My crown chakra also seemed to open wider. I asked The Source Ling Guang Calligraphy to open my spiritual channels fully. I feel much more clarity and light.

My regular five senses also seem to be much more sensitive. I felt as if I was receiving many gifts or downloads from Heaven. I am so very humbled and blessed. We are all extremely blessed.

M. D.
Ohio, U.S.A.

I have my life back after being a prisoner in my body

I got sick in 1995 but the doctor couldn't explain to me why I didn't recover. He told me I just had to live with it, but every year I felt worse. I had headaches and nausea. My liver hurt. I had eye problems and problems with mental clarity. And all of this became worse over time.

I tried many alternative healing methods without any relief. When I awoke on January 13, 2004 my whole body was in pain. It was hard to walk. My brain fog was intense. I couldn't go to work in that condition.

It was the first day of many years of lying in bed. No doctor could tell me what was wrong with me. All I knew was that my symptoms continued to worsen. My organs were slowly failing. It was hard to eat, hard to move, and hard to focus because of the brain fog and total lack of energy.

All I could do was lie down and stare at the ceiling. I was very sensitive to sound and movement. I couldn't concentrate and was completely disoriented at times, which made it very difficult to take care of myself or to go outside. I felt like I was captive inside my body and my house until I found a doctor who was willing to do some tests on my liver. Finally it was determined that my liver didn't detoxify as it should and many of the toxins were stored in my body—in my muscles, tissues, organs, nervous system, and brain.

After five years in bed fighting for my life, a new fight started. How could I get all the toxins out of my body? My body was so weak that it felt like it was too late.

On June 10, 2010 I went to a Free Soul Healing Evening with Dr. and Master Sha, and the next day I was very blessed to have a personal conversation with him. Master Sha said the main issue was the heavy soul blockages in my liver and that if nothing changed, my life could be deeply and drastically affected. Master Sha told me he could help me, but that it would take about two years before I could have my health back. I was so happy to have hope again.

I participated in as many teleconferences and webcasts as I could to learn the soul wisdom and practical techniques and to receive the blessings. I practiced every day for many hours. It was an intense period, but I could see and feel my inner organs starting to function again. I gained weight, the pain in my body decreased, and I felt how much love, care, and compassion there was for me. I was not just a number or a sick client. That was what really touched me.

After about two years, just like Master Sha said, there was a major break-through when I received Divine Services on September 11, 2012. My energy increased, my mental clarity improved, and the pain decreased.

It is now August 2013 and it is my first summer in ten years that I can enjoy the outside. I have started to work. I am doing physical exercise, taking long walks in nature. My social life is back, and I am so much stronger, healthier, and happier, and getting better every day. It really is a miracle to me.

I can never thank Master Sha, the Divine, Tao, and The Source enough for all that has been given to me and for saving my life.

Barbara Kuipers
Zandvoort, Netherlands

Practice. Practice. Practice.
Heal. Heal. Heal.
Heal your spiritual, mental, emotional, and physical bodies. Heal your spiritual, mental, emotional, and physical bodies. Heal your spiritual, mental, emotional, and physical bodies.
Prevent sickness. Prevent sickness. Prevent sickness.
Rejuvenate soul, heart, mind, and body. Rejuvenate soul, heart, mind, and body. Rejuvenate soul, heart, mind, and body.
Prolong life. Prolong life. Prolong life.
Transform relationships. Transform relationships. Transform relationships.
Transform finances and business. Transform finances and business. Transform finances and business.
Increase intelligence. Increase intelligence. Increase intelligence.
Open your spiritual channels. Open your spiritual channels. Open your spiritual channels.
Bring success in every aspect of life. Bring success in every aspect of life. Bring success in every aspect of life.
Benefit more. Benefit more. Benefit more.

All of the above are Soul Orders. They are modern mantras. Do not quickly go through them. Go back and chant them seriously one more time. These are the teachings of Da Tao zhi jian, The Big Way is extremely simple.

Open your heart and soul. Chant from your heart and soul. Apply these sacred mantras in your daily life.

Help yourself.

Help your loved ones.

Help humanity and all souls to pass through this difficult historical period.

Love you. Love you. Love you.

Thank you. Thank you. Thank you.

> *I love my heart and soul*
> *I love all humanity*
> *Join hearts and souls together*
> *Love, peace and harmony*
> *Love, peace and harmony*

Create Love Peace Harmony Universal Family.

> *Chanting chanting chanting*
> *Divine chanting is healing*
> *Chanting chanting chanting*
> *Divine chanting is rejuvenating*
> *Singing singing singing*
> *Divine singing is transforming*
> *Singing singing singing*
> *Divine singing is enlightening*
>
> *Humanity is waiting for divine chanting*
> *All souls are waiting for divine singing*
> *Divine chanting removes all blockages*
> *Divine singing brings inner joy*
> *Divine is chanting and singing*
> *Humanity and all souls are nourishing*

Humanity and all souls are chanting and singing
World love, peace, and harmony are coming
World love, peace, and harmony are coming
World love, peace, and harmony are coming

5

The Source Ling Guang (Soul Light) Calligraphies: The Source Jing Qi Shen Field for Healing the Spiritual, Mental, Emotional, and Physical Bodies

I have shared a lot of spiritual wisdom about the Soul Light Era in my earlier books. I will emphasize this important teaching again.

On August 8, 2003 the Divine held a meeting in Heaven and announced that the last universal era was ending and a new era, the Soul Light Era, would begin on that day. The last era was named *Xia Gu*. "Xia" means *lower* or *near*. "Gu" means *ancient*. "Xia Gu" (pronounced *shyah goo*) means *near ancient*. It is the era that began fifteen thousand years before August 8, 2003, and ended on that day.

Before Xia Gu was the *Zhong Gu* era. "Zhong" means *middle*. "Gu" means *ancient*. "Zhong Gu" (pronounced *jawng goo*) means *middle ancient*. It is the era that started approximately thirty thousand years ago and ended approximately fifteen thousand years ago.

Before Zhong Gu was *Shang Gu*. "Shang" means *upper* or *far*. "Gu" means *ancient*. "Shang Gu" (pronounced *shahng goo*) means *far ancient*. It is the era that lasted from about forty-five thousand years ago to about thirty thousand years ago.

Reincarnation is a universal law. Human beings reincarnate. Time reincarnates also. Time reincarnates on Mother Earth through a cycle of eras. Each era lasts fifteen thousand years.

On August 8, 2003 the Xia Gu era ended and the Shang Gu era returned. The current Shang Gu era will also last fifteen thousand years and then the Zhong Gu era will return. The next Zhong Gu era will also last fifteen thousand years. Then the next Xia Gu era will return. Time reincarnation repeats this cycle:

Shang Gu → Zhong Gu → Xia Gu → Shang Gu →
Zhong Gu → Xia Gu…

August 8, 2003 was the end of the most recent Xia Gu era and the start of the new Shang Gu era. This era is called the Soul Light Era. Mother Earth is in the Fourth Dimension during the Shang Gu era. Mother Earth is in the Third Dimension during the Zhong Gu and Xia Gu eras.

Saints in the last Shang Gu era had extraordinary abilities and created many soul healing miracles. Now Shang Gu has returned. Many soul healing miracles will appear again on Mother Earth because of the Fourth Dimension. The Fourth Dimension has much higher frequency, vibration, and soul power than the Third Dimension.

A "miracle" is something extraordinary, an object of wonder, astonishment, and awe. The Source is the Creator of Heaven, Mother Earth, humanity, and countless planets, stars, galaxies, and universes. The power of The Source cannot be explained in words or comprehended by thoughts. Miracle stories in the human realm are everyday stories for The Source.

In 2008 my soul was uplifted to The Source. I was chosen as the servant of humanity and The Source. I was given the honor and authority to offer permanent soul mind body healing and blessing treasures from The Source to humanity and all souls.

In June 2013 The Source gave me new power to create The Source Calligraphy for healing, blessing, and life transformation. Because this is the Soul Light Era, this calligraphy is named *The Source Ling Guang Calligraphy*. "Ling" means *soul*. "Guang" means *light*. Ling Guang Calligraphy means *soul light calligraphy*. Each calligraphy carries The Source Field. It connects with countless saints. It connects with countless Heaven's saints' animals. It carries countless Heaven, Divine, Tao, and The Source healing and blessing treasures. I have explained earlier that The Source Field is The Source jing qi shen. The Source jing qi shen could remove soul mind body blockages of sickness to create soul healing miracles.

I have written nine The Source Ling Guang Calligraphies to share with you and humanity in this book. Please refer to the insert near the end of this chapter.

The Source Ling Guang Calligraphy *Ling Guang—Soul Light*

The first Source Ling Guang Calligraphy I share in this chapter is *Ling Guang*. "Ling" means *soul*. "Guang" means *light*. See the calligraphy of *Ling Guang* in figure 17. Refer to the color insert near the end of this chapter.

The power and significance of The Source Ling Guang Calligraphy can be summarized as follows:

- It carries The Source jing qi shen.
- It carries The Source love, forgiveness, compassion, and light.
- It connects with countless saints and all kinds of spiritual fathers and mothers in Heaven and on Mother Earth.
- It carries countless Heaven's saints' animals.
- It carries countless treasures of Heaven, the Divine, Tao, and The Source.

How to Apply The Source Ling Guang Calligraphy

How do you use The Source Ling Guang Calligraphy to heal the spiritual, mental, emotional, and physical bodies? Apply the Four Power Techniques:

Body Power. There are three ways to apply Body Power with The Source Ling Guang Calligraphy:

- Put one palm on the page with the photo of The Source Ling Guang Calligraphy. Put your other palm on any part of the body that needs healing.
- Put the page with the photo of The Source Ling Guang Calligraphy on any part of the body that needs healing.
- Meditate with The Source Ling Guang Calligraphy.

Soul Power. Say *hello*:

Dear The Source Ling Guang Calligraphy,
I love you, honor you, and appreciate you.
You carry The Source jing qi shen.
You have the power to remove soul mind body blockages of my
*   sicknesses.*

Dear the saints, Heaven's saints' animals, and treasures from Heaven,
*   the Divine, Tao, and The Source connected with and carried within*
*   The Source Ling Guang Calligraphy,*
I love you, honor you, and appreciate you.
You have immeasurable power to heal me.
Please heal me.
Thank you.

Mind Power. Visualize Ling Guang (soul light) shining in the area where you want healing. It is best to visualize golden light or rainbow light in the area that needs healing.

Sound Power. Chant silently or aloud:

Ling Guang heals me. Thank you.
Ling Guang heals me. Thank you.
Ling Guang heals me. Thank you.
Ling Guang heals me. Thank you.

Golden light heals me. Thank you.
Golden light heals me. Thank you.
Golden light heals me. Thank you.
Golden light heals me. Thank you.

Rainbow light heals me. Thank you.
Rainbow light heals me. Thank you.
Rainbow light heals me. Thank you.
Rainbow light heals me. Thank you…

As you chant, keep your eyes closed. Visualize light shining brightly and transparently in the sickness area. If your Third Eye is open, you could see the light transforming the area for which you requested healing. The area could have appeared dark or gray but it could change to golden or rainbow light through The Source Ling Guang Calligraphy blessing.

When the light and transparency transform the sickness area, your sickness transforms on the spot. This is the secret, sacred soul healing power of The Source. It takes time for many people to adapt to the power from The Source Ling Guang Calligraphy.

If your Third Eye is open, you could see other light such as purple, crystal, or other colors. This calligraphy shines multiple colors of light, both visible and invisible. The light from The Source Ling Guang Calligraphy is so beautiful that it cannot be explained in words.

Shingles outbreak healed in three days with The Source Calligraphy blessing

I recently have been under quite a bit of stress due to financial issues. When under this level of stress in the past, I have had outbreaks of shingles. I have had outbreaks six different times. I usually get outbreaks on the right side of my body that can last up to six weeks, even with medication. I have been unable to walk at times due to the intense pain. About a week ago I had another outbreak and received The Source Calligraphy blessing from Master Ximena, one of Master Sha's Worldwide Representatives.

After the blessing, the pain went from an 8 to about a 3 or 4. I went to sleep that evening, and when I awoke it was about a 2. By the next day the pain was gone. The vesicles healed and I felt back to normal. I am very grateful for this healing from The Source Calligraphy and Master Ximena. I did not have to miss any time with my clients, which was a total blessing. I am very grateful to the Divine and Master Sha for these amazing blessings and gifts. This was a healing miracle on many levels! I am deeply grateful.

Debra Manning, R.N. L.Ac.
Phoenix, Arizona, U.S.A.

Whole neighborhood more calm and at peace

I would like to share a little about my experience with The Source Calligraphy that I was deeply honored to receive in Toronto. The only challenge is that I don't know where to begin and what words to use.

This treasure has helped me and many others, including my whole neighborhood, on so many levels that I truly don't know how to express my gratitude. The whole area where I live has become more calm and at peace. The blessings and the light that come from the Calligraphy are very powerful and beautiful. Quite often I get knocked out by the frequency. I receive guidance, healing on all levels, and just amazing support that I would never have dreamed of or expected. I am deeply grateful and truly honored to hold this treasure that I know can help, and does help, many souls. It is a privilege.

Thank you, dear Master Sha, for sharing something so precious with us. Thank you with all of my heart and soul.

With much love and the deepest gratitude,

M. P.
Victoria, British Columbia, Canada

How long do you need to practice? The Source guided me at this moment that in order to receive the maximum benefits from The Source Ling Guang Calligraphy, it is best to practice for at least ten minutes each time. Some people could receive great results in that time, even in seconds. Some people could feel no improvement in ten minutes. Even if you feel no improvement, it does not mean there is no change. With ten minutes or more of practice with The Source Ling Guang Calligraphy field, the jing qi shen of the sickness is transforming in every moment. The jing qi shen of the sickness transforms in various degrees, but it may take some time for you to notice improvement. Be patient. Continue to practice. You could feel improvement later.

Practice is the key. One has to practice. Sickness is due to soul mind body blockages. I emphasize again:

> Soul blockages are bad karma.
> Mind blockages include negative mind-sets, negative attitudes,
>   negative beliefs, ego, attachments, and more.
> Body blockages include energy blockages and matter blockages.

The Source Ling Guang Calligraphy carries The Source jing qi shen, which carries much higher frequency and vibration than the jing qi shen of a human being. It could remove soul mind body blockages quickly. For some people who have chronic or life-threatening conditions, the soul mind body blockages could be very heavy. It does take time to remove heavy soul mind body blockages. Therefore, you need to practice, practice, practice. Be confident, patient, and persistent.

In summary, to practice with The Source Ling Guang Calligraphy:

- Practice at least ten minutes each time. The longer you practice, the better.
- The more often you practice, the better.
- For chronic or life-threatening conditions, add all of your practice time together to total at least two hours per day.

Your physical response after practicing could be:

- Instant improvement in pain, stiffness, and other conditions.
- Little or no improvement. If you do not feel any improvement, it does not mean that there is no change within. As I explained

earlier, the jing qi shen of the condition has been transformed at different levels, but you must continue to practice.

- Apparent intensification of the condition. This is not a bad sign. It is the process of releasing soul mind body blockages. Continue to practice. Great improvement could be on the way.

Please stop reading and do the practice now. Choose one system, organ, part of the body, or health condition that needs healing. You can apply this healing anytime and anywhere. All of The Source Ling Guang Calligraphies are soul healing treasures that could create all kinds of soul healing miracles.

You can come back to any The Source Ling Guang Calligraphy in this book anytime to receive healing. The Source Ling Guang Calligraphies are priceless soul healing treasures to offer all kinds of soul healing for the spiritual, mental, emotional, and physical bodies. Use them more and more. Benefit from them more and more.

At the end of each healing, please remember to offer your gratitude by saying *Love you. Love you. Love you. Thank you. Thank you. Thank you.*

Gratitude and Forgiveness Practice

After every practice it is vital to do a short gratitude and forgiveness practice. This is the way to do it:

Dear Divine,
Dear Tao, The Source,
Dear The Source Ling Guang Calligraphy,
Dear all of the saints, Heaven's saints' animals, and Heaven's
   treasures within The Source Ling Guang Calligraphy,
I am extremely honored to receive your blessing.
Please forgive my ancestors and me for all of the mistakes that we
   have made in all lifetimes.
I deeply apologize for all of our mistakes.
I will serve others unconditionally to make others happier and
   healthier.

I will work together with humanity and all souls to create a Love
    Peace Harmony Universal Family.
Love you. Love you. Love you.
Thank you. Thank you. Thank you.

This short gratitude and forgiveness practice must be offered with sincerity from the bottom of your heart.

The Source Calligraphy comforts young child

Today I was standing in front of The Source Calligraphy for my daily medi-tation. It was 2 a.m. and the candles were burning calmly, giving a smooth light to the Calligraphy. When I focused on the Calligraphy, the words start-ed to clearly stand out in 3D. They grew very big and were moving closer to me. It was an impressive and beautiful sight.

A bit before 2 a.m., our little two-year-old son had awakened and started to cry and called out for his mum. My wife went to calm him and returned to sleep again.

During my meditation, I heard my son again several times starting to sob and cry out. Each time I right away asked The Source Calligraphy to serve him and comfort him. And each time he calmed down right away and did not cry for mum again. My wife was able to continue sleeping, our little sweetie was comforted, and I could continue my meditation.

I was very grateful.

Gerard R.
Canada

Heal and Prevent Unhealthy Conditions of the Four Extremities and Rejuvenate the Four Extremities

So many people have health challenges with the four extremities. In my teaching, all sickness is due to soul mind body blockages. The Source Ling Guang Calligraphy carries The Source Field, which could remove

soul mind body blockages for healing. If you do not have health challenges with the four extremities, the following practices could help you
prevent sickness in the four extremities and rejuvenate them.

I will also teach you three methods of applying The Source Ling
Guang Calligraphy and lead you to use them one by one to receive healing, prevention of sickness, and rejuvenation.

Three Methods to Practice with The Source Ling Guang Calligraphy

Method 1—Place One Palm on The Source Ling Guang Calligraphy

The first method is to place one palm on The Source Ling Guang
Calligraphy. Place the other palm on the organ, system, or part of the
body that needs healing.

HEAL AND PREVENT CONDITIONS OF THE HIPS AND REJUVENATE
THE HIPS WITH SOUL LIGHT

Apply the Four Power Techniques with The Source Ling Guang
Calligraphy to heal and rejuvenate the hips:

Body Power. Refer to the color insert near the end of this chapter.
Put one palm on figure 17, The Source Ling Guang Calligraphy *Ling
Guang*. Put your other palm on a hip.

Soul Power. Say *hello*:

> *Dear Divine,*
> *Dear Tao, The Source,*
> *Dear The Source Ling Guang Calligraphy* Ling Guang,
> *Dear countless saints, Heaven's saints' animals, and Heaven's*
>   *treasures within The Source Ling Guang Calligraphy* Ling
>   Guang,
> *I love you, honor you, and appreciate you.*
> *Please heal my hips, prevent unhealthy conditions in my hips, and*
>   *rejuvenate my hips.*
> *Thank you.*

Mind Power. Visualize soul light from The Source Ling Guang Calligraphy *Ling Guang* radiating and vibrating through your hips. Golden light or rainbow light would be good.

Sound Power. Chant silently or aloud:

> *The Source Ling Guang Calligraphy heals my hips, prevents unhealthy conditions in my hips, and rejuvenates my hips. Thank you.*
> *The Source Ling Guang Calligraphy heals my hips, prevents unhealthy conditions in my hips, and rejuvenates my hips. Thank you.*
> *The Source Ling Guang Calligraphy heals my hips, prevents unhealthy conditions in my hips, and rejuvenates my hips. Thank you.*
> *The Source Ling Guang Calligraphy heals my hips, prevents unhealthy conditions in my hips, and rejuvenates my hips. Thank you.*
> *The Source Ling Guang Calligraphy heals my hips, prevents unhealthy conditions in my hips, and rejuvenates my hips. Thank you.*
> *The Source Ling Guang Calligraphy heals my hips, prevents unhealthy conditions in my hips, and rejuvenates my hips. Thank you.*
> *The Source Ling Guang Calligraphy heals my hips, prevents unhealthy conditions in my hips, and rejuvenates my hips. Thank you…*

Please stop reading now. Continue to chant for at least ten minutes. Chant a few times a day. The longer you chant and the more often you chant, the better the results you could receive. If you have a chronic or life-threatening condition of the hips, chant for two hours or more per day. Add all of your practice time together to total at least two hours per day.

Now we need to offer gratitude and forgiveness. This is also a sacred practice. The more we offer gratitude and forgiveness from the heart, the faster we can receive soul healing miracles. Let us do it together:

Dear Divine,
Dear Tao, The Source,
Dear The Source Ling Guang Calligraphy,
Dear all of the saints, Heaven's saints' animals, and Heaven's
    treasures within The Source Ling Guang Calligraphy,
I am extremely honored to receive your blessing.
Please forgive my ancestors and me for all of the mistakes that we
    have made in all lifetimes related with my hip issues.
I deeply apologize for all of our mistakes.
I will serve others unconditionally to make others happier and
    healthier.
I will work together with humanity and all souls to create a Love
    Peace Harmony Universal Family.
Love you. Love you. Love you.
Thank you. Thank you. Thank you.
Hao! Hao! Hao!
Thank you. Thank you. Thank you.
Gong song. Gong song. Gong song.

HEAL AND PREVENT CONDITIONS OF THE KNEES AND REJUVENATE THE KNEES WITH GOLDEN LIGHT

Millions of people suffer from knee problems, including arthritis, swelling, stiffness, misalignment, injuries, and more. Many people undergo knee replacement and other kinds of knee surgery. All of these issues are due to soul mind body blockages.

Let us do a practice to heal and prevent unhealthy conditions of the knees and rejuvenate the knees.

Apply the Four Power Techniques with The Source Ling Guang Calligraphy *Ling Guang*:

Body Power. Put one palm on figure 17, The Source Ling Guang Calligraphy *Ling Guang*. Put your other palm on a knee. If you do not have knee issues, you will receive prevention of sickness and rejuvenation for your knees.

Soul Power. Say *hello*:

> *Dear Divine,*
> *Dear Tao, The Source,*
> *Dear The Source Ling Guang Calligraphy* Ling Guang,
> *Dear countless saints, Heaven's saints' animals, and Heaven's*
>   *treasures within The Source Ling Guang Calligraphy,*
> *I love you, honor you, and appreciate you.*
> *Please heal my knees, prevent unhealthy conditions in my knees, and*
>   *rejuvenate my knees.*
> *Thank you.*

Mind Power. Visualize golden light from The Source Ling Guang Calligraphy radiating and vibrating through your knees.

Sound Power. Chant silently or aloud:

> *Golden light from The Source Ling Guang Calligraphy heals and*
>   *rejuvenates my knees. Thank you.*
> *Golden light from The Source Ling Guang Calligraphy heals and*
>   *rejuvenates my knees. Thank you.*
> *Golden light from The Source Ling Guang Calligraphy heals and*
>   *rejuvenates my knees. Thank you.*
> *Golden light from The Source Ling Guang Calligraphy heals and*
>   *rejuvenates my knees. Thank you.*
> *Golden light from The Source Ling Guang Calligraphy heals and*
>   *rejuvenates my knees. Thank you.*
> *Golden light from The Source Ling Guang Calligraphy heals and*
>   *rejuvenates my knees. Thank you.*
> *Golden light from The Source Ling Guang Calligraphy heals and*
>   *rejuvenates my knees. Thank you…*

Please stop reading. Close your eyes and continue to chant and visualize for at least ten minutes.

Chant a few times a day. The longer you chant and the more often you chant, the better the results you could receive. If you have chronic or life-threatening conditions of the knees, chant for two hours or more per day. Add all of your practice time together to total at least two hours per day.

I would like to offer a brief teaching on chanting and why you need to close your eyes while you practice. To close your eyes is to help you visualize. In the previous healing practice, you visualized the brightest golden light radiating and vibrating in and around the knees. This is Mind Power and Yi Mi (Thinking Secret).

There are two ways to chant. One way is to chant out loud. This is yang chanting, which vibrates the bigger cells and spaces in the body. The other way is to chant silently. This is yin chanting, which vibrates the smaller cells and spaces. Both ways work. If you cannot chant aloud for any reason, chanting silently is absolutely fine.

At the end of every practice, remember to say silently three times, *Love you. Love you. Love you. Thank you. Thank you. Thank you.* This is to offer gratitude to The Source Ling Guang Calligraphy, which connects with all of the saints, Heaven's saints' animals, and Divine, Tao, and The Source treasures carried within The Source Ling Guang Calligraphy.

Remember to offer a gratitude and forgiveness practice:

Dear Divine,
Dear Tao, The Source,
Dear The Source Ling Guang Calligraphy Ling Guang,
Dear all of the saints, Heaven's saints' animals, and Heaven's
    treasures within The Source Ling Guang Calligraphy,
I am extremely honored to receive your blessing to heal and
    rejuvenate my knees.
Please forgive my ancestors and me for all of the mistakes that we
    have made in all lifetimes related to my knee challenges.
Dear all of the people and all the souls that my ancestors and I have
    harmed, hurt, and taken advantage of in the physical body and
    knees in all lifetimes,

I deeply apologize for all of the mistakes we have made.
I will serve others unconditionally to make others happier and
     healthier.
I will work together with humanity and all souls to create a Love
     Peace Harmony Universal Family.
Love you. Love you. Love you.
Thank you. Thank you. Thank you.

Divine Healing Hands in action

For the last two years, my mom has been suffering from knee pain due to osteoarthritis and it was progressively getting worse. Doctors suggested performing knee surgery. She was not keen on having surgery at the age of seventy. So, I started to offer her healing every morning during the daily Free Divine Healing Hands Blessings Teleconference. I live in Vancouver, British Columbia and my mom lives in Malaysia.

One day when I phoned my mom, she said that she had a "strange" story to share. In the middle of the night when she was sleeping, she was jolted awake after feeling someone's hands massaging her knees and "performing some kind of chiropractic adjustments" on both of her knees. She was startled because no one else was in the room with her and she was wondering whose "invisible hands" were on her knees. I asked her if she remembered what time that had happened. She said it was roughly 1 a.m. or 2 a.m. in Malaysia, which would have been around the time I was offering her remote Divine Healing Hands blessings! She said the next morning she woke up and had more strength in her knees and could get out of bed without any support. She could also go down the stairs without pain. We both felt very blessed and grateful that my mom actually physically felt Divine Healing Hands "in action"! It was a very special incident that moved and touched us deeply.

Not long after, Master Sha visited Vancouver in 2013 and started to offer Original Jing Qi Shen healing. I asked my mom to give soul healing a try before opting for surgery, which she was starting to consider seriously as the knee pain had returned and seemed to be aggravated. I gifted her Divine Knees and Original Jing Qi Shen for Knees and started chanting. Her knees started to heal progressively. Instead of surgery, my mom decided to try stem cell injection in the knee. With soul healing practices and the medical treatment, my mom is happy to regain her active life again completely free of knee pain. I feel so happy and grateful that I was able to help my mom despite the distance between us.

Thank you, Divine. Thank you, Master Sha. We are beyond grateful to Master Sha for the incredible soul healing wisdom and powers that continue to enrich and transform our lives.

D. L.
Vancouver, British Columbia, Canada

Eighteen years of knee pain healed: no limitations!

I met Master Sha in 2005 in New York. My husband had received major healing from Master Sha the month before in San Francisco, so we decided to drive to New York to attend an event with Master Sha there.

I was a nurse and had lupus for eighteen years before I met Master Sha. I had to retire because all my joints were so damaged from the disease. Doctors recommended knee replacement surgery on both knees because I have no cartilage in my knees.

Master Sha did a Soul Transplant for my knees to replace the souls of my knees. I immediately felt better. Prior to meeting Master Sha, my life was very limited. I could not go grocery shopping because I couldn't walk far enough. I could stand for only about fifteen minutes before I would have to sit down.

The day after I received the Soul Transplant, my husband and I spent all day sightseeing in New York City. I walked all over, sitting down only to eat lunch. My husband finally had to say slow down! I just wanted to keep going.

Three weeks later, we attended a wedding. I hadn't worn heels in many years because of my knee pain. I brought along a pair of flat shoes, thinking I would wear the heels to the church ceremony only. I not only wore my heels through the entire wedding and reception, I danced in them for about three hours without knee pain!

My lupus went into remission three years ago and now I have no limitations at all. I can play with my grandchildren. I can garden. I have no limitations. I am eternally grateful.

Diane G.
Salem, Oregon, U.S.A.

Method 2—Place The Source Ling Guang Calligraphy Directly on the Area That Needs Healing

Let me lead and guide you in the second way of applying The Source Ling Guang Calligraphy for healing, prevention of sickness, and rejuvenation.

I will emphasize again that the healing in this book is extremely simple, powerful, and beyond comprehension. Why? Every system, every organ, and every cell of the body is made of jing qi shen. When a person gets sick, the jing qi shen of the unhealthy area has been depleted or gone out of balance. The Source Ling Guang Calligraphy carries The Source Field, which is the jing qi shen of The Source. The jing qi shen of The Source can transform the jing qi shen of the unhealthy area. Therefore, healing could happen quickly, even instantly.

Let us apply the Four Power Techniques with The Source Ling Guang Calligraphy *Ling Guang* to continue to heal and prevent unhealthy conditions in the four extremities and rejuvenate the four extremities.

We will do a practice for healing and rejuvenating the shoulders.

HEAL AND PREVENT CONDITIONS OF THE SHOULDERS AND REJUVENATE THE SHOULDERS WITH RAINBOW LIGHT

Body Power. Hold the book and place the page with figure 17, The Source Ling Guang Calligraphy *Ling Guang*, on a shoulder that needs healing. If your shoulder does not need healing, you will receive prevention of sickness and rejuvenation.

Soul Power. Say *hello*:

> *Dear Divine,*
> *Dear Tao, The Source,*
> *Dear The Source Ling Guang Calligraphy,*
> *Dear countless saints, Heaven's saints' animals, and Heaven's*
>   *treasures within The Source Ling Guang Calligraphy,*
> *I love you, honor you, and appreciate you.*
> *Please heal and rejuvenate my shoulder.*
> *Thank you.*

Mind Power. Visualize rainbow light from The Source Ling Guang Calligraphy radiating and vibrating in and around your shoulder.

Sound Power. Chant silently or aloud:

> *Rainbow light from The Source Ling Guang Calligraphy heals and*
> *   rejuvenates my shoulder. Thank you.*
> *Rainbow light from The Source Ling Guang Calligraphy heals and*
> *   rejuvenates my shoulder. Thank you.*
> *Rainbow light from The Source Ling Guang Calligraphy heals and*
> *   rejuvenates my shoulder. Thank you.*
> *Rainbow light from The Source Ling Guang Calligraphy heals and*
> *   rejuvenates my shoulder. Thank you.*
> *Rainbow light from The Source Ling Guang Calligraphy heals and*
> *   rejuvenates my shoulder. Thank you.*
> *Rainbow light from The Source Ling Guang Calligraphy heals and*
> *   rejuvenates my shoulder. Thank you.*
> *Rainbow light from The Source Ling Guang Calligraphy heals and*
> *   rejuvenates my shoulder. Thank you...*

Stop reading. Chant and visualize for ten minutes. The longer you chant and the more often you chant, the better the results you could receive. If you have a chronic or life-threatening condition of the shoulder, chant for two hours or more per day. Add all of your practice time together to total at least two hours per day.

Now offer gratitude and forgiveness:

> *Dear Divine,*
> *Dear Tao, The Source,*
> *Dear rainbow light from The Source Ling Guang Calligraphy* Ling
> *   Guang,*
> *Dear all of the saints, Heaven's saints' animals, and Heaven's*
> *   treasures within The Source Ling Guang Calligraphy,*
> *I am extremely honored to receive your blessing to heal and*
> *   rejuvenate my shoulder.*

Please forgive my ancestors and me for all of the mistakes that we
     have made in all lifetimes related to challenges with my shoulder.
Dear all of the people and all the souls that my ancestors and I have
     harmed, hurt, and taken advantage of in the physical body and
     shoulders in all our lifetimes,
I deeply apologize for all of our mistakes.
I will serve others unconditionally to make others happier and
     healthier.
I will work together with humanity and all souls to create a Love
     Peace Harmony Universal Family.
Love you. Love you. Love you.
Thank you. Thank you. Thank you.

Heal and Prevent Conditions of the Elbows and Rejuvenate the Elbows with Purple Light

Many people suffer from conditions of the elbows, including tennis elbow, bursitis, tendinitis, injuries, and more. Do the following practice often to transform these conditions. If you do not have challenges with your elbows, you will receive prevention of sickness and rejuvenation.

Body Power. Place figure 17, The Source Ling Guang Calligraphy *Ling Guang*, on an elbow that needs healing.

Soul Power. Say *hello:*

Dear Divine,
Dear Tao, The Source,
Dear purple light of The Source Ling Guang Calligraphy Ling
     Guang,
Dear countless saints, Heaven's saints' animals, and Heaven's
     treasures within The Source Ling Guang Calligraphy,
I love you, honor you, and appreciate you.
Please heal and rejuvenate my elbow.
Thank you.

Mind Power. Visualize purple light from The Source Ling Guang Calligraphy shining in and around your elbow.

Sound Power. Chant silently or aloud:

> *Purple light from The Source Ling Guang Calligraphy heals and rejuvenates my elbow. Thank you.*
> *Purple light from The Source Ling Guang Calligraphy heals and rejuvenates my elbow. Thank you.*
> *Purple light from The Source Ling Guang Calligraphy heals and rejuvenates my elbow. Thank you.*
> *Purple light from The Source Ling Guang Calligraphy heals and rejuvenates my elbow. Thank you.*
> *Purple light from The Source Ling Guang Calligraphy heals and rejuvenates my elbow. Thank you.*
> *Purple light from The Source Ling Guang Calligraphy heals and rejuvenates my elbow. Thank you.*
> *Purple light from The Source Ling Guang Calligraphy heals and rejuvenates my elbow. Thank you…*

Stop reading. Continue to chant for ten minutes. You can also chant:

> *Purple light. Perfect elbow.*
> *Purple light. Perfect elbow.*
> *Purple light. Perfect elbow.*
> *Purple light. Perfect elbow.*
> *Purple light. Perfect elbow.*
> *Purple light. Perfect elbow.*
> *Purple light. Perfect elbow…*

Remember, the longer you chant and the more often you chant, the better the results you could receive. If you have a chronic or life-threatening condition of the elbow, chant for two hours or more per day. Add all of your practice time together to total at least two hours per day.

It is always important to offer gratitude and forgiveness. I cannot emphasize this enough. The more sincerely you offer gratitude and forgiveness, the faster you could be healed. Do not think this is repetitive. *This is the key to creating soul healing miracles.*

Let us do the gratitude and forgiveness practice:

> *Dear Divine,*
> *Dear Tao, The Source,*
> *Dear purple light from The Source Ling Guang Calligraphy* Ling Guang,
> *Dear all of the saints, Heaven's saints' animals, and Heaven's treasures within The Source Ling Guang Calligraphy,*
> *I am extremely honored to receive your blessing to heal and rejuvenate my elbow.*
> *Please forgive my ancestors and me for all the mistakes we have made in all lifetimes related to the condition of my elbow.*
> *Dear all of the people and all the souls that my ancestors and I have harmed, hurt, and taken advantage of in the physical body and elbows in all lifetimes,*
> *I deeply apologize for all of our mistakes.*
> *I will serve others unconditionally to make others happier and healthier.*
> *I will work together with humanity and all souls to create a Love Peace Harmony Universal Family.*
> *Love you. Love you. Love you.*
> *Thank you. Thank you. Thank you.*

Always remember:

> *Practice. Practice. Practice.*
> *Benefit from it. Benefit from it. Benefit from it.*
> *Create your own soul healing miracles.*

HEAL AND PREVENT CONDITIONS OF THE WRISTS AND HANDS AND REJUVENATE THE WRISTS AND HANDS WITH CRYSTAL LIGHT

Millions of people have issues with their wrists and hands, including arthritis, carpal tunnel syndrome, ganglion cysts, tendinitis, injuries, and more. Do the following practice often to heal your wrists and hands.

If you do not need healing, you will receive prevention of sickness and rejuvenation for your wrists and hands.

Body Power. Place figure 17, The Source Ling Guang Calligraphy *Ling Guang*, on a wrist and hand that need healing. If your wrist and hand do not need healing, you will receive prevention of sickness and rejuvenation. Do not skip the practice.

Soul Power. Say *hello*:

> *Dear Divine,*
> *Dear Tao, The Source,*
> *Dear crystal light of The Source Ling Guang Calligraphy* Ling Guang,
> *Dear countless saints, Heaven's saints' animals, and Heaven's*
>   *treasures within The Source Ling Guang Calligraphy,*
> *I love you, honor you, and appreciate you.*
> *Please heal and rejuvenate my wrist and hand.*
> *Thank you.*

Mind Power. Visualize crystal light from The Source Ling Guang Calligraphy *Ling Guang* vibrating in and around your wrist and hand.

Sound Power. Chant silently or aloud:

> *Crystal light from The Source Ling Guang Calligraphy heals*
>   *and rejuvenates my wrist and hand. Thank you . . .*

Then continue to chant:

> *Crystal light*
> *Crystal light*
> *Crystal light*
> *Crystal light*
> *Crystal light*
> *Crystal light*
> *Crystal light . . .*

Heal my wrist and hand. Thank you.
Heal my wrist and hand. Thank you.
Heal my wrist and hand. Thank you.
Heal my wrist and hand. Thank you.
Heal my wrist and hand. Thank you.
Heal my wrist and hand. Thank you.
Heal my wrist and hand. Thank you…

Stop reading. Continue to chant for ten minutes. The longer you chant each time, and the more times you practice each day, the better. There is no time limit. Practice as long as you can to restore your health to normal as quickly as possible. For serious or chronic conditions of the wrists and hands, chant for two hours or more per day. Add all of your practice time together to total at least two hours per day.

Now we need to express gratitude and forgiveness. Always remember to do this practice after every healing session. Silently invoke:

Dear Divine,
Dear Tao, The Source,
Dear crystal light from The Source Ling Guang Calligraphy,
Dear all of the saints, Heaven's saints' animals, and Heaven's
*   treasures within The Source Ling Guang Calligraphy,*
I am extremely honored to receive your blessing to heal and
*   rejuvenate my wrists and hands.*
Please forgive my ancestors and me for all of the mistakes we have made
*   in all lifetimes related to the challenges with my wrists and hands.*
Dear all of the people and all the souls that my ancestors and I have
*   harmed, hurt, and taken advantage of in the physical body and*
*   wrists and hands in all lifetimes,*
I deeply apologize for all of our mistakes.
I will serve others unconditionally to make others happier and
*   healthier.*
I will work together with humanity and all souls to create a Love
*   Peace Harmony Universal Family.*
Love you. Love you. Love you.
Thank you. Thank you. Thank you.

Method 3—Meditate with The Source Ling Guang Calligraphy

The third method of applying The Source Ling Guang Calligraphy is to meditate with it. Simply open this book to a photo of any The Source Ling Guang Calligraphy and connect with the saints, saints' animals, and treasures within the calligraphy. I will lead and guide you to do this in the next practice.

The methods I share in this book for healing, prevention of sickness, and rejuvenation are extremely simple. They could be too simple to believe. Do the practices anyway. You will experience the benefits.

An important sacred phrase from ancient spiritual teaching is:

If you want to know if a pear is sweet, taste it.

I would like to request of you and every reader, do not use your logical mind to make any judgments on the healing methods that I am sharing with you in this book and my previous books. What you need to do is *taste the pear*. Continue to practice. After ten minutes of practice, results could range from great improvement to little improvement to no improvement. If you feel better, you will believe right away that these methods work. If you do not feel better, please remember to have more patience and continue to practice. Some people have very heavy soul mind body blockages. Some people have taken medications for many years for their ailments. Some people suffer from chronic or life-threatening conditions. Do not expect instant soul healing miracles.

Practice more and more.
Be patient.
Be confident.
Trust.
I wish for you to receive a soul healing miracle or great results as soon as possible.

There is an ancient sacred teaching that has become more and more widely known:

Everyone and everything is divided into yin and yang.

For example, a physical eye and the Third Eye are a yin yang pair. The physical eye is the yang eye. The Third Eye is the yin eye. The physical eye sees the physical world, including a sunset, a television, this book, and much more. The Third Eye sees spiritual images of the Soul World.

Yin and yang can be subdivided endlessly. Those who have not opened their Third Eye cannot see spiritual images. Therefore, spiritual images are invisible to them.

Those who have an open Third Eye, especially those who have advanced Third Eye abilities, can see spiritual images very well. The spiritual images are visible to them.

However, spiritual images can be subdivided further into yin and yang aspects. There are always some spiritual images that cannot be seen even by someone with advanced Third Eye abilities. This is called *invisible light.*

Therefore, someone who has an open Third Eye can see light that a normal physical eye cannot see, but there is also some invisible light that someone with advanced Third Eye abilities still cannot see.

Now I am ready to release a major spiritual secret. The Source Field carries The Source light that is divided into visible light and invisible light. To see the visible light, one must have an open Third Eye. The invisible light cannot be seen even by one who has advanced Third Eye abilities.

Invisible light has a tinier, more refined vibration than visible light. Invisible light has higher frequency and more power to remove soul mind body blockages. The Source Ling Guang Calligraphies carry The Source Field, which contains both visible light and invisible light. This is the first time that I have shared this wisdom. Let us apply this sacred wisdom right away.

HEAL AND PREVENT CONDITIONS OF THE ANKLES AND FEET AND
REJUVENATE THE ANKLES AND FEET WITH INVISIBLE GOLDEN LIGHT

Millions of people suffer from conditions of the ankles and feet, including arthritis, plantar fasciitis, bunions, warts, sprains, injuries, and much more.

Let me lead and guide you to practice the third method of applying The Source Ling Guang Calligraphy, which is to meditate with it. If you do not need healing for your ankles and feet, they will receive prevention of sickness and rejuvenation.

Apply the Four Power Techniques and open this book to figure 17 with The Source Ling Guang Calligraphy *Ling Guang* and sit facing it.

Body Power. Sit up straight. There are three ways to sit. You may sit naturally in a chair. You may sit in the half-lotus position. You may sit in the full-lotus position. Keep your back free and clear; do not lean against the back of the chair or a wall. Place one palm on your lower abdomen below the navel. Place your other palm on an ankle or foot that needs healing.

Soul Power. Say *hello*:

> *Dear Divine,*
> *Dear Tao, The Source,*
> *Dear invisible golden light of The Source Ling Guang Calligraphy*
>   *Ling Guang,*
> *Please send your jing qi shen to my ankles and feet.*
> *Dear countless saints, Heaven's saints' animals, and Heaven's*
>   *treasures within The Source Ling Guang Calligraphy,*
> *I love you, honor you, and appreciate you.*
> *Please send your soul healing to my ankles and feet.*
> *Thank you.*

Mind Power. Visualize invisible golden light from The Source Ling Guang Calligraphy flowing to your ankles and feet.

Sound Power. Chant silently or aloud:

Invisible golden light of The Source Ling Guang Calligraphy heals
my ankles and feet. Thank you.
Invisible golden light heals me. Perfect ankles and feet.
Invisible golden light heals me. Perfect ankles and feet.
Invisible golden light heals me. Perfect ankles and feet.
Invisible golden light heals me. Perfect ankles and feet.
Invisible golden light heals me. Perfect ankles and feet.
Invisible golden light heals me. Perfect ankles and feet...

Chant for ten minutes. If you have a chronic condition, chant for two hours or more per day. The longer you chant and the more often you chant, the better the results you could receive. Add all of your practice time together to total at least two hours per day.

Always remember to offer gratitude and forgiveness after each practice:

Dear Divine,
Dear Tao, The Source,
Dear invisible golden light of The Source Ling Guang Calligraphy,
Dear all of the saints, Heaven's saints' animals, and Heaven's
treasures within The Source Ling Guang Calligraphy,
I am extremely honored to receive your blessing for my ankles and
feet.
Please forgive my ancestors and me for all of the mistakes we have
made in all lifetimes related to my ankles and feet.
Dear all of the people and all the souls that my ancestors and I have
harmed, hurt, and taken advantage of in the physical body and
ankles and feet in all lifetimes,
I deeply apologize for all our mistakes.
I will serve others unconditionally to make others happier and
healthier.
I will work together with humanity and all souls to create a Love
Peace Harmony Universal Family.
Love you. Love you. Love you.
Thank you. Thank you. Thank you.

Now I would like to share a story on the power of the The Source
Ling Guang Calligraphies.

Healing went far beyond the physical pain

*I was extremely honored to receive one of Master Sha's The Source Ling
Guang Calligraphies.*

*What happened was so amazing. I meditated with The Source Calligraphy
and requested healing blessings for the sharp pain that was constantly in my
left upper back. At the end of the meditation there was no pain. I cannot say
thank you enough.*

*I was also aware of the presence of many saints. They were healing and
rejuvenating me. As they were healing the physical aspect they were also
healing other aspects connected with the physical condition. They were
healing what had contributed to the physical condition as well as what had
resulted from it. These blessings were not limited just to me.*

Thank you. Thank you. Thank you.

M. M.
Redwood City, California, U.S.A.

Four of the Most Powerful Divine and Source Sacred Mantras

In my Soul Power Series books, I have taught readers all over the world
to chant four sacred phrases. They are actually four sacred mantras.
These mantras are the key secrets, wisdom, knowledge, and practical
techniques for creating soul healing miracles. These four sacred phrases
or mantras are:

Love melts all blockages and transforms all life.

Forgiveness brings inner joy and inner peace to all life.

**Compassion boosts energy, stamina, vitality,
and immunity of all life.**

**Light heals all sickness, prevents all sickness, transforms
relationships, transforms finances and business, increases
intelligence, opens spiritual channels,
and brings success to all life.**

These four sacred phrases are literally Heaven, Divine, and The
Source mantras. I will explain further.

Now chant *love melts all blockages and transforms all life* with me for
one minute:

> *Love melts all blockages and transforms all life.*
> *Love melts all blockages and transforms all life.*
> *Love melts all blockages and transforms all life.*
> *Love melts all blockages and transforms all life.*
> *Love melts all blockages and transforms all life.*
> *Love melts all blockages and transforms all life.*
> *Love melts all blockages and transforms all life…*

When you chant, chant from the bottom of your heart. Just speaking
the words is not enough. Chant with your heart. The most important
key is to connect with Heaven, the Divine, and Tao. Silently connect
with them before you chant. Do it like this:

> *Dear Heaven,*
> *Dear Divine,*
> *Dear Tao, The Source,*
> *I love you.*
> *My love and your love have a different frequency and vibration.*
> *Please bless me while I am chanting.*
> *I am very grateful.*

Now chant again, from your heart:

Love melts all blockages and transforms all life.
Love melts all blockages and transforms all life.
Love melts all blockages and transforms all life.
Love melts all blockages and transforms all life.
Love melts all blockages and transforms all life.
Love melts all blockages and transforms all life.
Love melts all blockages and transforms all life...

You can chant this mantra for healing any sickness. Choose one part of the body for healing and then invoke as follows:

Dear Heaven, Divine, and The Source mantras,
Please heal my _____ (name an area for which you are
    requesting healing).
Thank you.

Then chant:

Love melts all blockages and transforms all life.
Love melts all blockages and transforms all life.
Love melts all blockages and transforms all life.
Love melts all blockages and transforms all life.
Love melts all blockages and transforms all life.
Love melts all blockages and transforms all life.
Love melts all blockages and transforms all life...

Please stop reading, close your eyes, and continue to chant for ten minutes. After ten minutes of chanting, check how you feel. Continue to practice more and more to completely restore your health.

You may think that *love melts all blockages and transforms all life* is theory. I want to share with each of you that the theory *is* the practice. Theory and practice are two aspects, but they are two sides of the same coin. The most important wisdom is that they are One. It is just like yin and yang. Yin and yang are two aspects, but yin and yang are One.

I would like to share a one-sentence secret:

**The most important *theory* in spiritual practice
is the most important *practice*; they are One.**

For example, we are chanting *love melts all blockages and transforms all life*. This is theory, but it is the most important practice. Chanting *love melts all blockages and transforms all life* is one of the most important mantras for creating soul healing miracles.

Everything is made of jing qi shen. The word *love* carries jing qi shen. *Melts all blockages* carries jing qi shen. *Transforms all life* carries jing qi shen. *Love melts all blockages and transforms all life* also carries jing qi shen.

If you have advanced Third Eye abilities or if you have opened your advanced spiritual channels, you could see the soul of *love*. The soul of love is a light being. The soul of *melts all blockages* is another light being. The soul of *transforms all life* is another light being. When you chant *Love melts all blockages and transforms all life,* the light beings from this sacred phrase or mantra will transform your systems, organs, cells, DNA, and RNA. The frequency and vibration of your body, systems, organs, cells, DNA, and RNA will transform.

Why does chanting need to be repeated again and again? Because we need to continue to apply the frequency and vibration of love to continue to transform the frequency and vibration of our body, systems, organs, cells, DNA, and RNA. We need love's frequency and vibration to transform the frequency and vibration of our spiritual body, mental body, emotional body, and physical body. There is no time limit. Why do I always say, *Chant longer each time and chant more times each day*? Because the transformation of jing qi shen from our small, human love to the greatest love of the Divine and Tao takes time.

Why do I lead you to say, *Dear Heaven, Dear Divine, and Dear Tao*? Because Heaven's love, the Divine's love, and Tao's love have a much higher frequency and vibration than our human love. This is the way to practice:

Dear Heaven's love,
Please heal my _____ (choose any part of the body).
Thank you.

Then chant:

Love melts all blockages and transforms all life.
Love melts all blockages and transforms all life.
Love melts all blockages and transforms all life.
Love melts all blockages and transforms all life.
Love melts all blockages and transforms all life.
Love melts all blockages and transforms all life.
Love melts all blockages and transforms all life…

Continue to chant for ten minutes.

Love melts all blockages and transforms all life has power beyond words.

Heal and Prevent Conditions of the Neck and Rejuvenate the Neck

Place one palm on your neck and your other palm on your lower abdomen below the navel. This is Body Power. Put your mind on your neck and visualize light, which is Mind Power. Soul Power is to invoke the souls for healing. This is the way to do it:

Dear Heaven's love,
I deeply honor and appreciate you.
Please heal my neck.
Thank you.

To apply one of the Four Power Techniques is powerful. To apply all of the Four Power Techniques together is much more powerful. Continue to practice by applying the Four Power Techniques together.

Keep one hand on your neck. Your mind is still concentrating on visualizing light shining in your neck. You have invoked Heaven's love. Now add the last power, Sound Power.

Chant:

Heaven's love
Heaven's love
Heaven's love
Heaven's love

Heaven's love
Heaven's love
Heaven's love...

Chant *Heaven's love* from the bottom of your heart for ten minutes. Then check how your neck feels. I am sharing the sacred wisdom and practice by using this example of healing the neck. You can apply this sacred wisdom and practice to heal any part of the body. What I want to share with you and every reader again is Da Tao zhi jian: *The Big Way is extremely simple.*

Now choose another part of the body. Stop reading. Do not skip this part because the practices are the most important part of the book. I am leading you to practice through my instructions in the book. Please seriously do the practices to receive the greatest benefits.

I want to help you create soul healing miracles. How can we create soul healing miracles? We must learn the sacred wisdom and do the sacred practices. We have to practice. The practices are extremely simple. They could be too simple to believe, but do not skip the practices.

When my master and spiritual mentor Dr. and Master Zhi Chen Guo was still on Mother Earth, I asked him, "What is the biggest challenge to spreading soul healing?" He said, "The biggest challenge is that people find it hard to believe the simplicity and results of soul healing."

I would like to share a story with you.

Many years ago I taught a workshop in Toronto, Canada at the Learning Annex. A woman suffered from serious arthritis. One of her knees was very swollen. It was very difficult for her to walk. I taught, shared, and led all of the participants to chant for five to ten minutes, *I love my knee* or *I love my shoulder* according to their needs. About ten minutes later the woman stood up and walked without pain. As her tears flowed out, she said, "This is a miracle for me."

Just chant *Heaven's love, Heaven's love, Heaven's love, Heaven's love*... You can bring Heaven's love to any part of the body or to any aspect of your life. *Love melts all blockages and transforms all life.* I emphasize the message of the Soul Healing Miracle Series again:

I have the power to create soul healing miracles
to transform all of my life.

You have the power to create soul healing miracles
to transform all of your life.

Together we have the power to create soul healing miracles
to transform all life of humanity and all souls in Mother Earth
and countless planets, stars, galaxies, and universes.

Expand the wisdom and practice. You can apply this teaching for any healing and any life transformation. For example, you can say:

Dear Divine Love,
I cannot appreciate you enough.
I cannot honor you enough.
Please heal me.
Thank you.

Continue the healing for the part of the body that you requested earlier or choose another part of the body. Practice for another ten minutes.

Apply Tao Love in the same way. Tao is The Source. Tao Love is The Source love. Many people may still not be clear with the concept of The Source and the Divine. The Divine is the spiritual father or mother for humanity and all souls. Tao is The Source that creates Heaven, Mother Earth, and countless planets, stars, galaxies, and universes.

Now let me lead you to do soul healing for the emotional body. You have learned in chapters 2 and 4 that the physical organs and the emotional body are interconnected through the Five Elements. The liver connects with anger. The heart connects with depression and anxiety. The spleen connects with worry. The lungs connect with grief and sadness. The kidneys connect with fear.

If you have emotional imbalances of anger, depression, anxiety, worry, grief, sadness, or fear, do the following practices. If you do not have any of these emotional imbalances, you will receive prevention of these unbalanced emotions.

Heal Anxiety

Millions of people on Mother Earth suffer from anxiety. This practice could remove soul mind blockages that cause anxiety. If you do not have anxiety, this practice could serve you by preventing anxiety.

Body Power. Put one palm below the navel on your lower abdomen. Put your other palm over your heart. Remember, the heart is the authority organ of the Fire element, and is connected with anxiety in the emotional body.

Soul Power. Say *hello*:

> *Dear Tao love,*
> *I love you, honor you, and appreciate you.*
> *Please heal my anxiety.*
> *I am very grateful.*
> *Thank you.*

Mind Power. Visualize Ling Guang (soul light) shining in and around your heart.

Sound Power. Chant silently or aloud:

> *Tao love*
> *Tao love*
> *Tao love*
> *Tao love*
> *Tao love*
> *Tao love*
> *Tao love…*

Chant for ten minutes. Connect with Tao. Tao love carries the frequency and vibration of The Source that could remove the soul mind body blockages of your anxiety. This is how to heal anxiety to create your own soul healing miracle.

Always remember to offer gratitude and forgiveness:

> *Dear Tao love,*
> *I love you, honor you, and appreciate you.*
> *Your love can remove soul mind body blockages of my anxiety.*
> *I am extremely grateful.*
> *Please forgive my ancestors and me for all the mistakes we have*
> *made in all lifetimes related to anxiety.*
> *Dear all of the people and all the souls that my ancestors and I have*
> *harmed, hurt, and taken advantage of in the emotional body,*
> *including through anxiety and more in all lifetimes,*
> *Please forgive me.*
> *I will serve humanity, Mother Earth, and all souls unconditionally.*
> *Thank you.*

Then sing the Divine Soul Song *Love, Peace and Harmony*:[23]

> *Lu La Lu La Li*
> *Lu La Lu La La Li*
> *Lu La Lu La Li Lu La*
> *Lu La Li Lu La*
> *Lu La Li Lu La*
> *I love my heart and soul*
> *I love all humanity*
> *Join hearts and souls together*
> *Love, peace and harmony*
> *Love, peace and harmony*

Millions of people suffer from anxiety. I wish that everyone who suffers from anxiety would practice and create their own soul healing

---

[23] I received the *Divine Soul Song Love, Peace and Harmony* from the Divine on September 10, 2005. It is a powerful healing and blessing treasure that carries divine frequency and vibration with divine love, forgiveness, compassion, and light. You can download an mp3 file of *Love, Peace and Harmony* at www.LovePeaceHarmonyMovement.com. To chant this Divine Soul Song is to self-clear negative karma.

miracles. If you do not have anxiety, you can still do the practice. It will help you *prevent* anxiety.

The above teaching has shared with you and every reader the secrets, wisdom, knowledge, and practical techniques of *Love melts all blockages and transforms all life*. You could experience the teaching of love and the practice of love in many parts of my book. Do not think this is redundant. We cannot apply love enough.

The Source Ling Guang Calligraphy *Da Ai—Greatest Love*

The second The Source Ling Guang Calligraphy I share in this chapter is *Da Ai*. "Da" means *big*. "Ai" means *love*. "Da Ai" (pronounced *dah eye*) means *greatest love*.

Da Ai is the greatest love. Da Ai is unconditional love. There are some people who cannot offer unconditional love. There are some people who can only offer limited love. There are some people who cannot offer love at all. There are some people who cannot receive love. For example, some people have been abused. Their heart has been hurt or wounded. They cannot open to receive love or give love. This could develop into self-love issues or other issues.

This Source Ling Guang Calligraphy *Da Ai* could help with issues of self-love beyond words. Apply the teachings here and practice often. It could create all kinds of soul healing miracles.

Practice the same way as I explained with The Source Ling Guang Calligraphy *Ling Guang*.

Please stop reading and practice now.

Heal Depression

Apply The Source Ling Guang Calligraphy *Da Ai* (*dah eye*) with the Four Power Techniques together to heal depression.

Body Power. Refer to the color insert near the end of this chapter. Put one palm on the page with The Source Ling Guang Calligraphy *Da Ai* and one palm on the heart. (See figure 18.) The heart is the authority organ of the Fire element, which connects with depression in the emotional body.

Soul Power. Say *hello*:

> *Dear Divine,*
> *Dear Tao, The Source,*
> *Dear The Source Ling Guang Calligraphy* Da Ai,
> *Your unconditional love and greatest love can melt all blockages and*
>   *transform all life.*
> *I need Da Ai to open my heart and soul.*
> *Please remove soul mind body blockages of my depression.*
> *I am extremely honored and blessed.*
> *Dear all saints, Heaven's saints' animals, and treasures within this*
>   *calligraphy,*
> *I love you, honor you, and appreciate you.*
> *Please heal my depression.*
> *I am so grateful.*
> *Thank you.*

Mind Power. Visualize your heart shining Da Ai, which is *greatest love*. For this healing we are visualizing invisible rainbow light from the calligraphy.

Sound Power. Chant silently or aloud:

> *Invisible rainbow light of Da Ai melts all blockages and heals my*
>   *depression. Thank you.*
> *Invisible rainbow light heals my depression. Thank you.*
> *Invisible rainbow light heals my depression. Thank you.*
> *Invisible rainbow light heals my depression. Thank you.*
>
> *Da Ai opens my heart and soul. Thank you.*
> *Da Ai opens my heart and soul. Thank you.*
> *Da Ai opens my heart and soul. Thank you.*
> *Da Ai opens my heart and soul. Thank you.*
>
> *Da Ai allows me to receive love and offer love unconditionally.*
>   *Thank you.*

*Da Ai allows me to receive love and offer love unconditionally.
Thank you.
Da Ai allows me to receive love and offer love unconditionally.
Thank you.
Da Ai allows me to receive love and offer love unconditionally.
Thank you . . .*

Continue to chant:

*Da Ai
Da Ai
Da Ai
Da Ai
Da Ai
Da Ai
Da Ai*

*Da Ai invisible rainbow light
Da Ai invisible rainbow light
Da Ai invisible rainbow light
Da Ai invisible rainbow light
Da Ai invisible rainbow light
Da Ai invisible rainbow light
Da Ai invisible rainbow light . . .*

Stop reading and chant for ten minutes or longer. If you have a chronic or life-threatening condition, chant for two hours or more per day. The longer you chant and the more often you chant, the better the results you could receive. Add all of your practice time together to total two hours or more per day.

Now offer gratitude and forgiveness:

*Dear Divine,
Dear Tao, The Source,
Dear invisible rainbow light from The Source Ling Guang
Calligraphy Da Ai,*

Dear all of the saints, Heaven's saints' animals, and Heaven's
    treasures within The Source Ling Guang Calligraphy Da Ai,
I am extremely honored to receive your blessing to open my heart
    and soul to receive love and express love unconditionally and
    transform my depression.
Please forgive my ancestors and me for all of the mistakes that we
    have made in all lifetimes.
Dear all of the people and all the souls that my ancestors and I have
    harmed, hurt, and taken advantage of in the emotional body,
    including through depression and more in all lifetimes,
I deeply apologize for all of our mistakes.
Please forgive me.
I will serve others unconditionally to make others happier and
    healthier.
I will work together with humanity and all souls to create a Love
    Peace Harmony Universal Family.
Thank you. Thank you. Thank you.

I wish you great success in healing depression. Remember to practice, practice, practice.

Living a fulfilled life

There are many forms of miracles: healing miracles, life-saving miracles, finding one's true love, mending and transforming a challenged relationship, improved finances, and much more. The most profound miracle in my life is knowing that my life is guided after meeting and studying with Dr. and Master Zhi Gang Sha.

This guidance is a gentle voice that I hear from my Message Center (heart chakra) or a sense of knowing from time to time that helps me make decisions or follow a course of action. I feel at peace with my life, protected and blessed to move towards my highest destiny. I am transformed by Master Sha's teachings, blessings, and transmitted divine treasures. Before, I felt powerless and insignificant. It seemed that human suffering, so immense, could not be relieved by any level of commitment and undertaking. Now I feel that service is the most natural thing to do, and I am glad that I can serve in almost every moment. Whether through my intentions, through chanting, through healing blessings, or through meditation, whether at work or at rest, I can be of service to myself, others, my community, humanity, Mother Earth, and all universes. It is a joy to serve in this way without expectation; the rest is up to the Divine.

I am blessed by Master Sha and the Divine to have a loving family relationship. With the Da Ai Mi Zhou treasure that I received recently, I developed a deep love towards myself and my fellow brothers and sisters. My life is being nourished and blessed beyond words. My life is being guided. I am so grateful that I can serve in so many ways. This is my Soul Healing Miracle: the miracle of living a fulfilled life!

C. T.
Colfax, California, U.S.A.

Connecting with Heaven

I was so honored to have received one of Master Sha's Ling Guang Calligraphies. Every time I begin my meditation with the scroll, the letters quickly appear to become pure light. They begin to shine brightly and I feel like I enter into the scroll and travel with great speed to the other side. I often land in different places. Last time I meditated, I asked that my soul, heart, and mind be purified.

In my last three meditations, I saw Shi Jia Mo Ni Fo (the founder of Buddhism) with me. This time he took me to the land of golden buddhas. It was a golden land with golden light and many golden buddhas. I entered a golden temple. The temple was very tall with pointed rooftops. Inside the temple, I sat and meditated. There were saints dancing, humming, and singing. They appeared and disappeared. Two saints appeared around me and offered me teachings.

One of them removed my heart and purified it with light and replaced it in my body. The other one made an incision on my backside from the back of my neck along my spinal column and removed a black snake from inside me and replaced it with a golden snake.

Another saint appeared in front of me. I was told to study as they showed me Heaven's scroll with Heaven's messages. I was told that as Master Sha wrote scrolls for Mother Earth, he also wrote scrolls for Heaven and they are practicing with those scrolls just as we are.

I was told that I needed further purification, and my soul was taken and plunged into what I thought was the ocean, but it was an ocean made up of the universe, stars, and shiny objects. It was exquisite. I don't recall much more than this as I was in deep meditation, came back, and fell asleep.

I am forever grateful for this beautiful experience. I feel more connected to the heavens and more purified from this experience.

N. M.
Mumbai, India

Heal Grief

I will lead you to apply The Source Ling Guang Calligraphy *Da Ai* with the Four Power Techniques to heal grief.

Body Power. Place the page with figure 18, The Source Ling Guang Calligraphy *Da Ai*, on your lungs. The lungs in the physical body and grief in the emotional body are interconnected.

Soul Power. Say *hello*:

> *Dear The Source Ling Guang Calligraphy* Da Ai,
> *Dear bright white light of The Source Ling Guang Calligraphy* Da Ai,
> *Dear all saints, all saints' animals, and all treasures from Heaven, the Divine, Tao, and The Source within the Da Ai Calligraphy,*
> *I love you, honor you, and appreciate you.*
> *Please heal my lungs and, in my emotional body, grief.*
> *Thank you.*

Mind Power. Visualize bright white light shining in your lungs.

Sound Power. Chant silently or aloud:

Da Ai Calligraphy heals my grief. Thank you.
Da Ai Calligraphy heals my grief. Thank you.
Da Ai Calligraphy heals my grief. Thank you.
Da Ai Calligraphy heals my grief. Thank you.

Da Ai Calligraphy heals my grief. Thank you.
Da Ai Calligraphy heals my grief. Thank you.
Da Ai Calligraphy heals my grief. Thank you…

Bright white light
Bright white light
Bright white light
Bright white light
Bright white light
Bright white light
Bright white light…

Continue to chant for ten minutes. If you have grief or sadness, be sure to chant for a minimum of ten minutes each time you practice. If you have chronic grief or sadness, chant for two hours or more per day. The longer you chant and the more often you chant, the better the results you could receive. Add all of your practice time together to total at least two hours per day.

The Source Ling Guang Calligraphy *Da Kuan Shu—Greatest Forgiveness*

The third Source Ling Guang Calligraphy I share in this chapter is *Da Kuan Shu*. "Da" means *greatest*. "Kuan Shu" means *forgiveness*. "Da Kuan Shu" (pronounced *dah kwahn shoo*) means *greatest forgiveness*.

Millions of people have heard or read about the healing abilities of Jesus. When Jesus said, "You are forgiven," miracle healing happened. Jesus offered divine forgiveness. In my personal opinion, Jesus offered Divine Karma Cleansing when he said, "You are forgiven."

Human beings have made mistakes in all lifetimes, including killing, harming, taking advantage of others, stealing, lying, cheating, and more. In some spiritual teachings throughout history this has been known as "sin." To be forgiven is to be forgiven for one's sins from this lifetime and past lifetimes. It is different terminology, but it is karma cleansing.

Master Peter Hudoba, one of my top teachers, Disciples, and Worldwide Representatives, shares his story:

I met Master Sha for the first time on October 14, 2000.

I was solemnly quiet on the ride from the airport to his house. After some initial brief exchanges upon my arrival, we settled down in his living room to have a cup of tea.

Master Sha asked me, "Why did you come to see me?"

I answered, "Master Sha, there is some evil force that is destroying my life."

Master Sha's reply was very short: "There is no evil force; it is you. It is your karma; the result of your past life mistakes that keep coming back to you."

I understood. I asked Master Sha, "What can I do to dissolve this karma?"

He replied, "Ask God to forgive you."

That seemed too simple to me. From my years of Buddhist studies I knew what karma was. I also knew that millions of monks spent their whole lives in monasteries practicing daily to clear their negative karma, and still could not succeed.

I thought, "How could simply asking God to forgive me be enough?"

Yet, deep inside, I had deep reverence for Master Sha and I remembered his advice very well. And when the appropriate time came and I had reached that special state of being totally sorry for all that I had ever done wrong, I asked God to forgive me.

It was then that the issues that had been blocking me for so long began to dissolve.

I am so grateful in my heart to Master Sha and Heaven.

In the last few years I have offered one of the most important and powerful teachings in the Soul Power Series. This teaching is Forgiveness Practice. Doing Forgiveness Practice regularly is vital to transform blockages, including issues with health, emotions, relationships, finances, business, and much more. How does it work? Negative karma is the soul's record of unpleasant services from all lifetimes, current and past. Forgiveness Practice is key to self-clearing karma to remove blockages in every aspect of life.

Before we practice with the Source Ling Guang Calligraphy *Da Kuan Shu,* I will share with you a heart-touching story about Forgiveness Practice.

In 2012 I was in Frankfurt, Germany. I held a meeting with a few of my top students in Europe. They sincerely did Forgiveness Practice with one another. Each one faced another, looked into each other's eyes, sincerely asked for forgiveness from, and offered unconditional forgiveness to the other. They also asked Heaven, the Divine, and The Source, as well as any souls they or their ancestors had harmed in any lifetime, to forgive them. In addition, they offered unconditional forgiveness to all souls who had harmed their ancestors and them in this lifetime and past lifetimes. Everyone was deeply touched and moved by this practice.

I did a spiritual reading with Heaven and was extremely surprised by the impact this practice had. It was so powerful. Thirty percent of the relationship karma among them from all lifetimes was cleared just by doing this sincere Forgiveness Practice. The students were very touched, and understood deeply the power of forgiveness and the importance of Forgiveness Practice.

In my teaching, forgiveness brings inner joy and inner peace. I strongly encourage you to do regular Forgiveness Practice to transform every aspect of life.

I cannot emphasize enough, when you apply The Source Ling Guang Calligraphy *Da Kuan Shu,* sincerely apologize from the bottom of your heart for all of the mistakes that your ancestors and you have made in all lifetimes.

Let us continue to do Forgiveness Practice. Apply the Four Power Techniques:

Body Power. Place your left palm over your sternum and Message Center (heart chakra) and your right hand in the traditional prayer position, with fingers pointing upward. This new prayer position for the Soul Light Era is a special signal and connection with Heaven. It is a Shen Mi (Body Secret) for universal service. It is also named the Soul Light Era Universal Service Hand Position and the Soul Light Era Hands Shen Mi. (See figure 19.)

Soul Power. Say *hello*:

> *Dear Divine,*
> *Dear Tao, The Source,*
> *Please forgive my ancestors and me for all of the mistakes that we*
>   *have made in all of our lifetimes, including all past lifetimes and*
>   *this lifetime.*

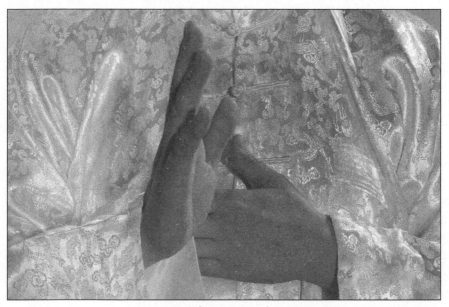

FIGURE 19. Soul Light Era Prayer Position

In order to be forgiven, I will offer unconditional universal service to humanity and all souls.
Thank you.

Unconditional universal service includes all kinds of activities, behaviors, speech, and thoughts that make others happier and healthier. Unconditional universal service is service without asking for anything in return. It is selfless service. Many of you do volunteer work. You may serve children, the poor, the homeless, spiritual groups, hospitals, disaster areas, and more without asking for anything in return. You may donate money to charities and causes. This is all wonderful and important service. To chant mantras and meditate is also important service because it brings love, forgiveness, compassion, and light from Heaven to humanity and all souls.

Heaven includes healing angels, archangels, ascended masters, saints, buddhas, bodhisattvas, gurus, lamas, kahunas, and all kinds of spiritual fathers and mothers from all traditions and belief systems, the Divine, Tao, and The Source.

Return to the practice, and then chant the Divine Soul Song *Love, Peace and Harmony*.

Heaven guided me to create the Love Peace Harmony Movement to form the Love Peace Harmony Universal Family. There are approximately one million people on Mother Earth who chant or listen to the Divine Soul Song *Love, Peace and Harmony*. I have given this beautiful and heart-touching Divine Soul Song as a gift to humanity. I have relinquished the copyright. You can download this Divine Soul Song as an mp3 file from my website, www.drsha.com. Sing this Divine Soul Song as much as you can to remove blockages and transform every aspect of your life.

How does the Divine Soul Song *Love, Peace and Harmony* work? Divine Soul Songs carry divine frequency and vibration, with divine love, forgiveness, compassion, and light. Divine frequency and vibration can transform the frequency and vibration of your health, emotions, relationships, finances, and more.

Mind Power. Visualize golden or rainbow light from the Divine and The Source shining among you and all the souls that you and your ancestors have hurt or harmed in all lifetimes.

Love and forgiveness are the golden keys to unlock all gates of all life. Love melts all blockages and transforms all life. Forgiveness can self-clear karma to bring inner joy and inner peace to all life.

The fourth Power Technique is **Sound Power.** Let us chant or sing *Love, Peace and Harmony*:

> *Lu La Lu La Li*
> *Lu La Lu La La Li*
> *Lu La Lu La Li Lu La*
> *Lu La Li Lu La*
> *Lu La Li Lu La*
>
> *I love my heart and soul*
> *I love all humanity*
> *Join hearts and souls together*
> *Love, peace and harmony*
> *Love, peace and harmony*

This is a master mantra of the Divine. There is no time limit on how long to chant this Divine Soul Song. You could chant from morning to night. Play the CD of this song in your home, bedroom, workplace, or car. Have this Divine Soul Song playing 24/7 to create a divine feng shui field to offer healing blessings to all life. I will share one story with you now.

A gynecologist in India shared this story. Her father is a general surgeon. He suffered a stroke and collapsed in the operating room while performing surgery. Three days later he became blind in one eye. It was a very serious stroke. Half of his body was paralyzed. His daughter played the CD of *Love, Peace and Harmony* nonstop and silently requested that her father be healed. Her father was in the hospital. She played the CD at home. She applied the Soul Power technique, one of the Four Power Techniques. She said *hello*. She played the CD and silently said:

> *Dear Divine Soul Song* Love, Peace and Harmony,
> *I love you, honor you, and appreciate you.*
> *Please offer soul healing to my father.*
> *Thank you.*

Soul healing is quantum healing; it is not limited by distance or time. The Divine Soul Song created a divine field. The divine field carried divine frequency and vibration with divine love, forgiveness, compassion, and light to heal her father. It removed soul mind body blockages of her father's conditions.

A soul healing miracle happened. Her father recovered extremely quickly for such a serious condition. Every day her father improved. Within three weeks, he returned to work as a surgeon. His doctors were shocked by his recovery.

Thousands of soul healing miracles have been created through this Divine Soul Song. It is a priceless treasure that can create countless soul healing miracles for humanity. Please chant and listen to this Divine Soul Song more. I wish soul healing miracles can happen for you and your loved ones through this Divine Soul Song.

Remember, love and forgiveness are two of the most important practices. They are One. If you truly have love, you can forgive. If you can truly forgive, you have love. To chant the Divine Soul Song *Love, Peace and Harmony* is to practice divine love and divine forgiveness. The gynecologist's father received soul healing miracles through the Divine Soul Song because the Divine Soul Song carries divine love and divine forgiveness, which removed soul mind body blockages of her father's conditions. Therefore, her father received a heart-touching healing miracle in a very short time. Love is forgiveness. Forgiveness is love.

Let us now continue with Forgiveness Practice.

Chant silently:

> *Divine Forgiveness*
> *Divine Forgiveness*

Divine Forgiveness
Divine Forgiveness
Divine Forgiveness
Divine Forgiveness
Divine Forgiveness...

Invoke and connect with all souls that your ancestors and you have hurt, harmed, or taken advantage of in all lifetimes. Ask them to forgive you and your ancestors for your mistakes of harming them. Also tell them that you forgive them unconditionally if they have harmed you in any way in this lifetime and in past lifetimes.

Then chant:

I forgive you.
You forgive me.
Bring love, peace, and harmony.

I forgive you.
You forgive me.
Bring love, peace, and harmony.

I forgive you.
You forgive me.
Bring love, peace, and harmony.

I forgive you.
You forgive me.
Bring love, peace, and harmony...

Chant as much as you can. Chant for at least ten minutes per time. The more often and the longer you chant, the better.

Heal Anger

Now let us practice forgiveness by applying The Source Ling Guang Calligraphy *Da Kuan Shu* (figure 20) to heal anger.

Apply the Four Power Techniques:

Body Power. Place one palm gently on the photograph of The Source Ling Guang Calligraphy *Da Kuan Shu* (figure 20). Place your other palm over the liver. The liver connects with anger in the emotional body. If you do not have anger, this practice will prevent sickness in and rejuvenate your liver and prevent anger.

Soul Power. Say *hello*:

> *Dear Divine,*
> *Dear Tao, The Source,*
> *Dear The Source Ling Guang Calligraphy* Da Kuan Shu,
> *Dear all of the saints, Heaven's saints' animals, and Heaven's*
>   *treasures within The Source Ling Guang Calligraphy* Da Kuan
>   Shu,
> *I love you, honor you, and appreciate you.*
> *Please forgive my ancestors and me for all the mistakes we have*
>   *made in all lifetimes related to the liver and anger.*
> *I am very honored that I can receive forgiveness from all of you.*
> *Dear all souls who have hurt, harmed, or taken advantage of me and*
>   *my ancestors in this lifetime and in past lifetimes, I forgive you*
>   *unconditionally.*
> *Thank you.*

Mind Power. Open your eyes to look at the calligraphy or close your eyes to connect with the calligraphy. Visualize light from the calligraphy and Heaven coming to your liver area in order to remove the soul mind body blockages of anger.

Sound Power. Chant silently or aloud:

Da Kuan Shu (pronounced *dah kwahn shoo*) *heals my anger. Thank*
   you.
Da Kuan Shu heals my anger. Thank you.
Da Kuan Shu heals my anger. Thank you.
Da Kuan Shu heals my anger. Thank you.
Da Kuan Shu heals my anger. Thank you.
Da Kuan Shu heals my anger. Thank you.
Da Kuan Shu heals my anger. Thank you…

Greatest forgiveness heals my anger. Thank you.
Greatest forgiveness heals my anger. Thank you.
Greatest forgiveness heals my anger. Thank you.
Greatest forgiveness heals my anger. Thank you.
Greatest forgiveness heals my anger. Thank you.
Greatest forgiveness heals my anger. Thank you.
Greatest forgiveness heals my anger. Thank you…

Stop reading and chant for ten minutes now. The more often you
chant and the longer you chant, the better the results you could receive.
   Now we need to offer gratitude:

Dear Divine,
Dear Tao, The Source,
Dear The Source Ling Guang Calligraphy Da Kuan Shu,
Dear all of the saints, Heaven's saints' animals, and Heaven's
   treasures within The Source Ling Guang Calligraphy Da Kuan
   Shu,
I am extremely honored to receive your blessing.
I will serve others unconditionally to make others happier and
   healthier.
Dear all of the people and all the souls that my ancestors and I have
   harmed, hurt, and taken advantage of in the emotional body,
   including through anger and more in all lifetimes,
I will work together with humanity and all souls to create a Love
   Peace Harmony Universal Family.
Thank you. Thank you. Thank you.

You can apply The Source Ling Guang Calligraphy *Da Kuan Shu* for healing any challenge in the spiritual body, mental body, emotional body, or physical body. There is no limit for healing from The Source Ling Guang Calligraphy *Da Kuan Shu* or any Source Ling Guang Calligraphy because they are The Source Field. The power of The Source Field cannot be expressed enough by words or comprehended by thoughts. They carry the frequency and vibration of The Source with The Source love, forgiveness, compassion, and light that can transform the frequency and vibration of anyone and anything. We are extremely blessed.

The power of forgiveness and the power of The Source Ling Guang Calligraphies are beyond comprehension. Here is one person's experience meditating with her Source Ling Guang Calligraphy.

Blessing beyond comprehension

I love my morning meditation with The Source Ling Guang Calligraphy.

It is essential for raising my vibration to higher and higher frequencies at a speed beyond imagination and comprehension. It is enhancing my field by billions of times.

To start each day with such high vibration, and the experience of this magnificent field, is a blessing beyond description and comprehension.

I am extremely grateful.

Rulin Xiu, Ph.D.
Pahoa, Hawaii, U.S.A.

Heal Resentment, Bitterness, Hatred, Revenge, and Envy

Millions of people have challenges with not being able to forgive. The root cause for conflict between people, organizations, nations, and more is karma. Many people find it very hard to forgive others. Therefore, there are many issues among people such as resentment, bitterness, hatred, revenge, and envy. To hold any of these can cause conflict, unrest, fighting, and wars, as well as imbalances in the spiritual, mental, emotional, and physical bodies.

How to resolve all of these issues arising from the inability to forgive? Love and forgiveness are the golden keys to resolve them. Da Ai (pronounced *dah eye*) means *greatest love*. Da Kuan Shu (pronounced *dah kwahn shoo*) means *greatest forgiveness*. When beloved Jesus said, "You are forgiven," miracles happened. People who suffered major sickness carried serious soul mind body blockages. Jesus offered divine forgiveness. Therefore, miracles happened.

Like Jesus, our beloved Guan Yin, Bodhisattva of Compassion and Goddess of Grace, has created many soul healing miracles. What have Jesus and Guan Yin done? They have offered divine unconditional love and forgiveness, regardless of what mistakes a person has made to others. Jesus and Guan Yin's miracle healing have proven their Da Ai and Da Kuan Shu (*greatest love* and *greatest forgiveness*) to the Divine and Tao.

Why do we need to learn from Jesus, Guan Yin, and many other great teachers, including saints, buddhas, bodhisattvas, ascended masters, healing angels, archangels, lamas, gurus, kahunas, and many other spiritual fathers and mothers? It is because their Da Ai and Da Kuan Shu are examples for humanity. I would like to share a one-sentence secret with all readers and humanity:

**Da Ai and Da Kuan Shu (*greatest love and greatest forgiveness*)
are the golden keys to unlock all life.**

Apply The Source Ling Guang Calligraphies *Da Ai* and *Da Kuan Shu* with the Four Power Techniques to heal and prevent resentment, bitterness, hatred, revenge, and envy:

Body Power. Sit up straight with your back away from the chair. Connect with The Source Ling Guang Calligraphies *Da Ai* and *Da Kuan Shu.*

Soul Power. Say *hello*:

> *Dear The Source Ling Guang Calligraphy Da Ai,*
> *Dear The Source Ling Guang Calligraphy Da Kuan Shu,*
> *Dear invisible rainbow light of The Source Da Ai Calligraphy,*
> *Dear invisible rainbow light of The Source Da Kuan Shu*
>   *Calligraphy,*
> *Dear all saints, saints' animals, and treasures from the Divine and*
>   *The Source connected to and within The Source Ling Guang*
>   *Calligraphy Da Ai and The Source Ling Guang Calligraphy Da*
>   *Kuan Shu,*
> *I love you, honor you, and appreciate you all.*
> *You have the power to open my heart and soul in order to transform*
>   *all of the soul mind body blockages related with resentment,*
>   *bitterness, hatred, revenge, envy, and more.*
> *I deeply apologize for any resentment, bitterness, hatred, revenge,*
>   *envy, and more that my ancestors and I have carried in all*
>   *lifetimes.*
> *I am extremely honored that The Source has created The Source Ling*
>   *Guang Calligraphies Da Ai and Da Kuan Shu and that these*
>   *priceless treasures could remove soul mind body blockages of*
>   *resentment, bitterness, hatred, revenge, envy, and more.*
> *I am beyond grateful.*
> *Thank you.*

Mind Power. Visualize The Source Da Ai and Da Kuan Shu Calligraphies shining invisible rainbow light to your whole body, from head to toe, skin to bone.

Sound Power. Chant silently or aloud:

> *Da Ai (pronounced dah eye) Calligraphy heals me. Thank you.*
> *Da Ai Calligraphy heals me. Thank you.*
> *Da Ai Calligraphy heals me. Thank you.*
> *Da Ai Calligraphy heals me. Thank you.*

Da Kuan Shu (pronounced dah kwahn shoo) Calligraphy heals me.
   Thank you.
Da Kuan Shu Calligraphy heals me. Thank you.
Da Kuan Shu Calligraphy heals me. Thank you.
Da Kuan Shu Calligraphy heals me. Thank you.

Invisible rainbow light heals me. Thank you.
Invisible rainbow light heals me. Thank you.
Invisible rainbow light heals me. Thank you.
Invisible rainbow light heals me. Thank you.

All saints, saints' animals, and Heaven's treasures heal me. Thank
   you.
All saints, saints' animals, and Heaven's treasures heal me. Thank
   you.
All saints, saints' animals, and Heaven's treasures heal me. Thank
   you.
All saints, saints' animals, and Heaven's treasures heal me. Thank
   you...

Chant for ten minutes without stopping. There is no time limit. The
more you chant, the better.

Now I will offer an important teaching.

The Source Ling Guang Calligraphies carry and connect with countless saints, saints' animals, Heaven, the Divine, Tao, The Source, and
countless treasures within. As you read this book, practice with The
Source Ling Guang Calligraphies for at least ten minutes per time. If
you could practice for much longer than ten minutes per time, I would
be very happy for you. If you could practice many times a day, I would
be very happy for you.

The important teaching I am offering is that you can connect with the
saints, saints' animals, and Heaven's treasures within the calligraphies
anywhere and at any time. You can connect remotely.

For example, when you are walking you can silently invoke as
follows:

Soul Power. Say *hello*:

> *Dear The Source Ling Guang Calligraphy* Da Ai,
> *Dear The Source Ling Guang Calligraphy* Da Kuan Shu,
> *Dear invisible rainbow light of The Source Ling Guang Calligraphy*
>   Da Ai,
> *Dear invisible rainbow light of The Source Ling Guang Calligraphy*
>   Da Kuan Shu,
> *Dear all saints, saints' animals, and treasures from the Divine*
>   *and The Source connected to and carried within The Source*
>   *Ling Guang Calligraphy* Da Ai *and The Source Ling Guang*
>   *Calligraphy* Da Kuan Shu,
> *I love you, honor you, and appreciate you all.*
> *Please remove soul mind body blockages of resentment, bitterness,*
>   *hatred, revenge, envy, and more. Heal them and prevent them from*
>   *returning.*
> *I am extremely honored and humbled.*
> *Thank you.*

Mind Power. As you walk, visualize the invisible rainbow light shining and vibrating in your body from head to toe, skin to bone.

Sound Power. Chant silently or aloud:

> *Dear The Source Ling Guang Calligraphy* Da Ai,
> *Dear The Source Ling Guang Calligraphy* Da Kuan Shu,
> *Dear invisible rainbow light,*
> *Dear all saints, saints' animals, and treasures carried within and*
>   *connected with the calligraphies,*
> *Please heal me. Please heal me. Please heal me.*
> *I am extremely grateful.*
> *Thank you.*

Keep chanting during your walk.
Remember this one-sentence secret:

You can connect to The Source Ling Guang Calligraphy anywhere, anytime for healing and transforming all life.

I will share a story with you:

This morning, July 31, 2013 I awoke and my whole body and shoulders were very heavy and felt as though a weight was on them. I also experienced some heavy pressure on my head. A variety of emotions came up within me. One hour later, I was on the train and I connected remotely with my Tao Source Ling Guang Calligraphy and asked for a blessing. Within two minutes, all of the pain disappeared and I fell asleep on the train. When I awoke, we were at the next stop and I was free of pain and totally healed.

I cannot emphasize and appreciate the power of The Source Ling Guang Calligraphy enough. Thank you, Master Sha, for creating this Source Ling Guang Calligraphy for helping humanity. I am extremely grateful.

A. G.
Toronto, Canada

The Source Ling Guang Calligraphy *Da Ci Bei—Greatest Compassion*

Now we will practice with the fourth calligraphy in this chapter: The Source Ling Guang Calligraphy *Da Ci Bei.*

"Da" means *greatest.* "Ci Bei" means *compassion.* "Da Ci Bei" (pronounced *dah sz bay*) means *greatest compassion.*

Compassion boosts energy, stamina, vitality, and immunity of all life. It carries power beyond imagination.

The Source Ling Guang Calligraphy *Da Ci Bei* carries The Source Field of Source compassion. We will practice to receive the greatest benefits from The Source Compassion Field.

I will share a few stories about our beloved Guan Yin, the Bodhisattva of Compassion. She made a vow to help anyone on Mother Earth who calls her name. There are many miracle stories in history about Guan

Yin's unconditional service. These are soul healing miracle stories. Her soul created these miracles.

I will share one story in Chinese history.

Many fishermen lived in the southern part of China. They worked on a fishing boat and encountered a big storm at sea. The boat overturned and the men fell into the water. They called out, "Guan Yin, jiu ming." "Jiu ming" (pronounced *jeo ming*) means *save life*. After calling Guan Yin's name, they plummeted deeper into the water and lost consciousness. Before losing consciousness they thought they would surely die. They awoke some time later on shore. Their lives had been saved. Guan Yin's soul brought their physical bodies to the shore.

There are many other miracles stories created by Guan Yin's great compassion. People with chronic or life-threatening conditions have chanted *Qian Shou Qian Yan Da Ci Da Bei Guan Shi Yin Pu Sa* with great results. "Qian" means *thousand*. "Shou" means *hands*. "Yan" means *eyes*. "Da" means *big*. "Ci Bei" means *compassion* or *kindness*. "Pu Sa" means *bodhisattva*.

Qian Shou Qian Yan Da Ci Da Bei Guan Shi Yin Pu Sa (pronounced *chyen sho chyen yen dah sz dah bay gwahn shr yeen poo sah*) means *thousand soul hands, thousand soul eyes, big compassion, kindness, Guan Yin bodhisattva.* People who have been very sick with life-threatening conditions have had their health restored by chanting this mantra from the heart. There are countless heart-touching, moving, and life-saving stories about Guan Shi Yin Pu Sa. Billions of people in history have honored her.

Guan Yin sees and hears the suffering of humanity and serves unconditionally. Guan Yin is a great example of an unconditional servant who offers unconditional love, unconditional forgiveness, and unconditional compassion. This is the key message we need to learn from her. If humanity could offer unconditional love, forgiveness, and compassion to each other, humanity would be very different. Mother Earth would be very different.

I am deeply honored to be a lineage holder of Guan Yin. I have offered Guan Yin's permanent thousand soul hands and thousand soul eyes healing and blessing treasures to more than fifty people on Mother Earth to create the next generation of Guan Yin's lineage. Guan Yin and her lineage have decided that I could offer this honor to one thousand people on Mother Earth. Anyone who receives this priceless treasure becomes a lineage holder of Guan Yin. To receive a thousand soul hands and a thousand soul eyes in order to become a lineage holder is to become a better servant for humanity. We are blessed. Humanity is blessed.

In the last few years, the Divine and Tao asked me to teach that compassion boosts energy, stamina, vitality, and immunity of all life. Compassion has immeasurable power to heal all kinds of sickness. The Divine and Tao gave me the honor and authority to create The Source Ling Guang Calligraphy *Da Ci Bei* (*greatest compassion*).

Now we are ready to experience the power of greatest compassion. I have created The Source Ling Guang Calligraphy *Da Ci Bei* to serve each of you, dear readers, and your loved ones.

Boost Energy, Stamina, Vitality, and Immunity to Form a Jin Dan

Everyone can benefit from greater energy, stamina, vitality, and immunity. Apply the Four Power Techniques with The Source Ling Guang Calligraphy *Da Ci Bei* to boost energy, stamina, vitality, and immunity:

Body Power. Refer to the color insert near the end of chapter 5. Put one palm on figure 21, The Source Ling Guang Calligraphy *Da Ci Bei*. Put your other palm below the navel on your lower abdomen. The source of a human being's energy, stamina, vitality, and immunity is below the navel. This is ancient sacred teaching.

Soul Power. Say *hello*:

> *Dear Divine,*
> *Dear Tao, The Source,*
> *Dear The Source Ling Guang Calligraphy* Da Ci Bei,
> *Dear the saints, Heaven's saints' animals, and Heaven, Divine, and*
>   *Tao Source treasures within the calligraphy,*
> *I love you, honor you, and appreciate you.*
> *Please boost my energy, stamina, vitality, and immunity.*
> *Thank you.*

Mind Power. Visualize golden light from the calligraphy and from Heaven, Mother Earth, the Divine, and Tao pouring into your body from 360° to form a golden light ball inside your lower abdomen below your navel.

Sound Power. Chant silently or aloud:

> *Da Ci Bei* (pronounced *dah sz bay*) *boosts my energy, stamina, vitality, and immunity by forming a Jin Dan* (golden light ball) *in my lower abdomen. Thank you.*
> *Da Ci Bei boosts my energy, stamina, vitality, and immunity by forming a Jin Dan in my lower abdomen. Thank you.*
> *Da Ci Bei boosts my energy, stamina, vitality, and immunity by forming a Jin Dan in my lower abdomen. Thank you.*
> *Da Ci Bei boosts my energy, stamina, vitality, and immunity by forming a Jin Dan in my lower abdomen. Thank you.*
> *Da Ci Bei boosts my energy, stamina, vitality, and immunity by forming a Jin Dan in my lower abdomen. Thank you.*
> *Da Ci Bei boosts my energy, stamina, vitality, and immunity by forming a Jin Dan in my lower abdomen. Thank you.*
> *Da Ci Bei boosts my energy, stamina, vitality, and immunity by forming a Jin Dan in my lower abdomen. Thank you...*

Close your eyes when you chant. Visualize golden light from The Source Ling Guang Calligraphy *Da Ci Bei* pouring into your body from 360°. Totally relax. This light forms a golden light ball, which is the Jin Dan, in your lower abdomen. This Jin Dan is vital for boosting energy, stamina, vitality, and immunity. This Jin Dan is also vital for healing and preventing all kinds of sickness, rejuvenation, and prolonging life.

I cannot emphasize enough the importance of this exercise. Please bookmark this page. Come back to this page many times to do this practice. My advice is to do a thirty-minute practice per time. If you can do one hour, even better. The longer you practice and the more often you practice, the better. Continue with the same visualization or simply chant:

Form my Jin Dan; grow my Jin Dan.
Form my Jin Dan; grow my Jin Dan.
Form my Jin Dan; grow my Jin Dan.

Form my Jin Dan; grow my Jin Dan.
Form my Jin Dan; grow my Jin Dan.
Form my Jin Dan; grow my Jin Dan.
Form my Jin Dan; grow my Jin Dan…

Always remember to offer gratitude for the blessings received and do Forgiveness Practice:

> *Dear Divine,*
> *Dear Tao, The Source,*
> *Dear The Source Ling Guang Calligraphy* Da Ci Bei,
> *Dear all of the saints, Heaven's saints' animals, and Heaven's treasures*
>   *within The Source Ling Guang Calligraphy* Da Ci Bei,
> *I am extremely honored to receive your blessing to boost my energy,*
>   *stamina, vitality, and immunity by forming and growing my Jin*
>   *Dan.*
> *Please forgive my ancestors and me for all the mistakes we have made*
>   *in all lifetimes.*
> *I deeply apologize for all of our mistakes.*
> *I will serve others unconditionally to make others happier and*
>   *healthier.*
> *I will work together with humanity and all souls to create a Love*
>   *Peace Harmony Universal Family.*
> *Thank you. Thank you. Thank you.*

The Source Ling Guang Calligraphy can heal and bless any aspect of life, including nature and much more. Following is a story about a Source Ling Guang Calligraphy and flowers.

Dearest Beloved Master Sha,
I cannot thank you enough for The Source Ling Guang Calligraphy. I am so honored to have one. I have a small but powerful miracle I would like to share.
I bought some roses when I returned home from the retreat. I put three on my altar, below The Source Ling Guang Calligraphy, and six in my living room.

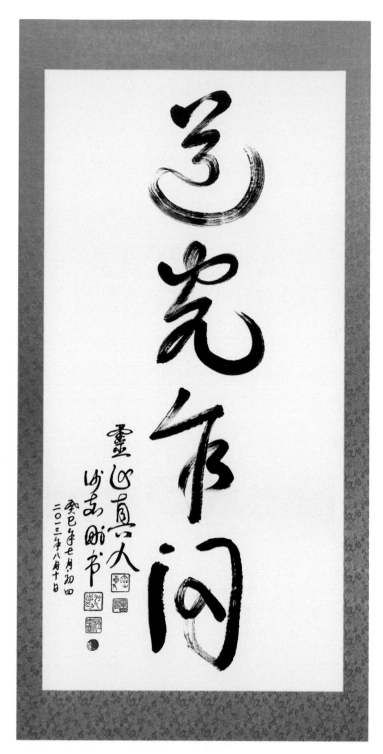

FIGURE 13
The Source Ling Guang Calligraphy Tao Guang Zha Shan

FIGURE 15

The Source Ling Guang Calligraphy Hei Heng Hong Ha

嘿哼了嗏唅

靈山真人沙志助书

癸巳年七月初四
二○二三年八月十日

光亮好美

灵山真人

河东助书

癸巳年七月初四

二〇一三年八月十日

FIGURE 17
The Source Ling Guang Calligraphy Ling Guang

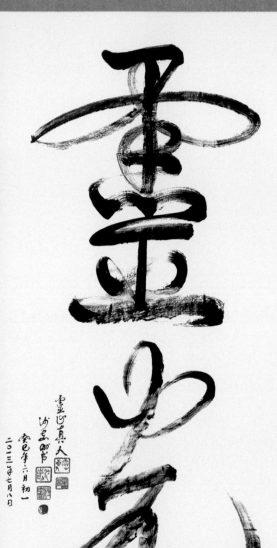

靈光

靈巴真人
沙彥 □节
二〇一三年七月八日
癸巳年六月初一

FIGURE 18
The Source Ling Guang Calligraphy Da Ai

F<small>IGURE</small> 18
The Source Ling Guang Calligraphy Da Ai

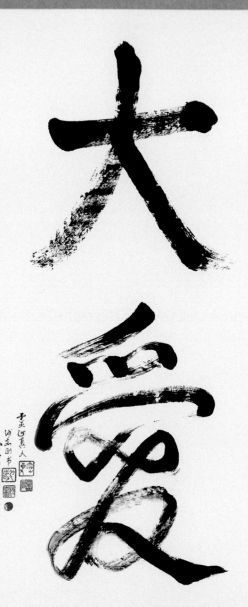

FIGURE 20
The Source Ling Guang Calligraphy Da Kuan Shu

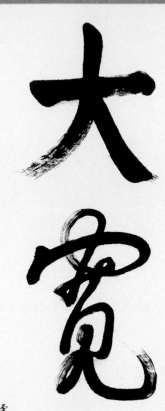

大寬宏

靈巴真人
沙泉阁书
癸巳年六月十五日
二〇一三年七月二十二日

FIGURE 21
The Source Ling Guang Calligraphy Da Ci Bei

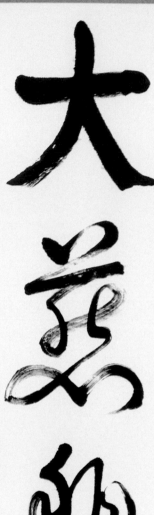

大慈悲

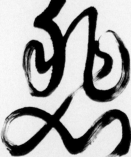

靈山真人
沙石所書
癸巳年六月十五日
二〇一三年七月二十二日

FIGURE 23
The Source Ling Guang Calligraphy Da Guang Ming

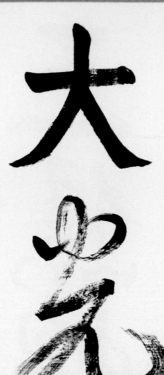

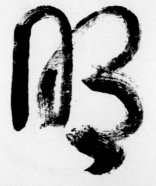

靈山真人
少玉敬书
癸巳年六月十五日
二〇一三年七月二十二日

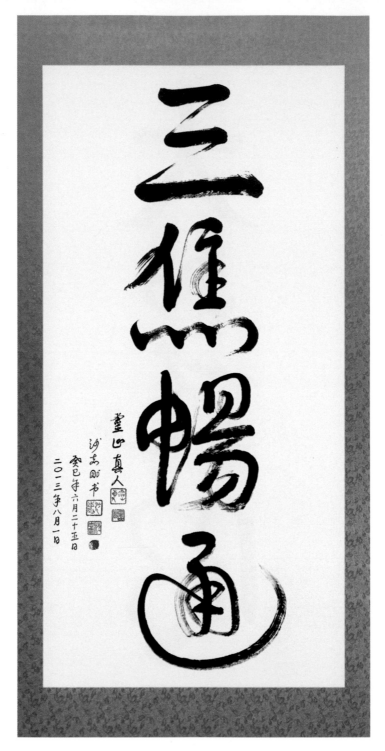

FIGURE 24
The Source Ling Guang Calligraphy San Jaio Chang Tong

The roses on the altar are spectacular. They look more beautiful than when I bought them. The roses in my living room have already wilted—living proof of the power of The Source Ling Guang Calligraphy. (See figure 22.)
With love and Total GOLD,[24]

S. Z.
Tucson, Arizona, U.S.A.

The Source Ling Guang Calligraphy *Da Ci Bei* could boost your energy, stamina, vitality, and immunity anytime and anywhere. To create soul healing miracles everyone needs powerful energy, stamina, vitality, and immunity. This Source Field of The Source Compassion is not only for boosting energy, stamina, vitality, and immunity; it is also a soul healing miracle treasure for all life. Apply this calligraphy for healing all unhealthy conditions. It also is the priceless treasure to form and grow your Jin Dan.

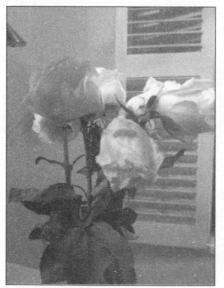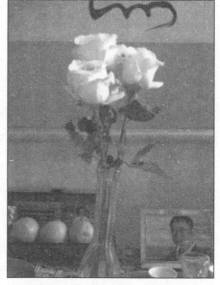

FIGURE 22. Roses in bloom

---

[24] Total GOLD means total gratitude, obedience, loyalty, and devotion to the Divine.

I wish for you to have powerful energy, stamina, vitality, and immunity.

I wish for you to form and grow your Jin Dan.

I wish for you to receive great soul healing miracles or results.

The Source Ling Guang Calligraphy *Da Guang Ming*— *Greatest Light*

Now we will practice with the fifth calligraphy in this chapter: The Source Ling Guang Calligraphy *Da Guang Ming*.

"Da" means *greatest*. "Guang Ming" means *light*. "Da Guang Ming" (pronounced *dah gwahng ming*) means *greatest light*.

Light heals the spiritual, mental, emotional, and physical bodies; prevents all sickness; purifies and rejuvenates soul, heart, mind, and body; transforms relationships; transforms business and finances; increases intelligence; opens spiritual channels; and brings success to every aspect of life.

Da Guang Ming is not ordinary light. It is the *greatest light*. The Source Ling Guang Calligraphy *Da Guang Ming* carries jing qi shen of the greatest light from The Source to transform the jing qi shen of your health, emotions, relationships, finances, business, intelligence, and every aspect of life. The power of Da Guang Ming for healing and blessing is beyond words and comprehension.

Heal Worry

Now let us practice with The Source Ling Guang Calligraphy *Da Guang Ming* (pronounced *dah gwahng ming*) for healing worry.

Apply the Four Power Techniques:

Body Power. Refer to the color insert near the end of this chapter. Sit in a chair with your back free and clear. Place one palm on figure 23, The Source Ling Guang Calligraphy *Da Guang Ming*. Place your other palm over the spleen (located on the left side of the body under the ribs).

Five thousand years ago, the scholars of traditional Chinese medicine revealed the connection between the spleen and worry in the emotional body. This means that worry can cause unhealthy conditions within the spleen, and sickness of the spleen can cause worry.

Soul Power. Say *hello*:

> *Dear Divine,*
> *Dear Tao, The Source,*
> *Dear The Source Ling Guang Calligraphy* Da Guang Ming,
> *Dear visible and invisible golden light of The Source Ling Guang*
>   *Calligraphy* Da Guang Ming,
> *Dear the saints, Heaven's saints' animals, and Heaven, Divine, Tao,*
>   *and Source treasures within the calligraphy,*
> *I love you, honor you, and appreciate you.*
> *Please heal my spleen and worry.*
> *Thank you.*

Mind Power. Visualize visible and invisible golden light from the calligraphy and from Heaven, Mother Earth, the Divine, and Tao pouring into your spleen from 360° to remove soul mind body blockages of worry. If you do not suffer from worry, you will receive prevention of sickness and rejuvenation of your spleen as well as prevention of worry.

Sound Power. Chant silently or aloud:

> *Visible and invisible golden light Da Guang Ming* (pronounced *dah*
>   *gwahng ming*) *heal my spleen and worry. Thank you.*
> *Visible and invisible golden light Da Guang Ming heal my spleen and*
>   *worry. Thank you.*
> *Visible and invisible golden light Da Guang Ming heal my spleen and*
>   *worry. Thank you.*
> *Visible and invisible golden light Da Guang Ming heal my spleen and*
>   *worry. Thank you.*
> *Visible and invisible golden light Da Guang Ming heal my spleen and*
>   *worry. Thank you.*
> *Visible and invisible golden light Da Guang Ming heal my spleen and*
>   *worry. Thank you.*
> *Visible and invisible golden light Da Guang Ming heal my spleen and*
>   *worry. Thank you...*

You can also continue to chant:

Da Guang Ming (pronounced *dah gwahng ming*)
Da Guang Ming
Da Guang Ming
Da Guang Ming
Da Guang Ming
Da Guang Ming
Da Guang Ming...

Continue to chant:

Golden light
Golden light
Golden light
Golden light
Golden light
Golden light
Golden light...

Please stop reading now and practice for at least ten minutes. The longer you can practice per time and the more often you practice, the better. For chronic or life-threatening conditions, chant for two hours or more per day. Add all of your practice time together to total two hours or more per day.

Now let us offer gratitude and forgiveness. Always remember to offer gratitude and forgiveness after every healing session.

Thank you, Divine.
Thank you, Tao, The Source.
Thank you, the Source Field, The Source Ling Guang Calligraphy Da
   Guang Ming.
Thank you, visible and invisible light from the calligraphy.
Thank you, all of the saints, saints' animals, and Heaven, Divine,
   and Tao treasures connected to and carried within the calligraphy.

*Please forgive my ancestors and me for all the mistakes we have
    made in all lifetimes related with the spleen and worry.*
I am extremely grateful for all of your blessings.
*Dear all of the people and all the souls that my ancestors and I have
    harmed, hurt, and taken advantage of in the emotional body,
    including through worry and more in all lifetimes,*
Please forgive me.
Thank you. Thank you. Thank you.

Heal Fear

Now let us practice with The Source Ling Guang Calligraphy *Da
Guang Ming* to heal fear. In traditional Chinese medicine and Five
Elements theory, kidneys in the physical body connect with fear in the
emotional body.

Apply the Four Power Techniques:

Body Power. Sit up with your back free, clear, and straight. Connect
with The Source Ling Guang Calligraphy *Da Guang Ming*.

Soul Power. Say *hello*:

> *Dear The Source Ling Guang Calligraphy* Da Guang Ming,
> *Dear all of the saints, saints' animals, and treasures of Heaven,
>   Divine, and Tao connected to and carried within The Source Ling
>   Guang Calligraphy* Da Guang Ming,
> *Dear bright blue light from The Source Ling Guang Calligraphy* Da
>   Guang Ming,
> *I love you, honor you, and appreciate you all.*
> *Please remove soul mind body blockages of my kidneys and heal my
>   fear.*
> *Thank you.*

Mind Power. Visualize bright blue light shining in your kidneys.

Sound Power. Chant silently or aloud:

> *Da Guang Ming Calligraphy* (pronounced *dah gwahng ming*)
> *Da Guang Ming Calligraphy*
> *Da Guang Ming Calligraphy*
> *Da Guang Ming Calligraphy*
> *Da Guang Ming Calligraphy*
> *Da Guang Ming Calligraphy*
> *Da Guang Ming Calligraphy . . .*

Continue to chant:

> *Greatest blue light*
> *Greatest blue light*
> *Greatest blue light*
> *Greatest blue light*
> *Greatest blue light*
> *Greatest blue light*
> *Greatest blue light . . .*

Stop reading and chant for at least ten minutes. The more you chant, the better the results you could experience. Remember, for chronic or life-threatening conditions, chant two hours or more per day. Add all of your practice time together to total at least two hours.

Let us show our gratitude and do Forgiveness Practice:

> *Dear Divine and Tao,*
> *Please forgive my ancestors and me for all of the mistakes that we*
>   *have made in all lifetimes related with fear and the kidneys.*
> *Dear all of the people and all the souls that my ancestors and I have*
>   *harmed, hurt, and taken advantage of in the emotional body,*
>   *including through fear and more in all lifetimes,*
> *Please forgive me.*
> *I will serve unconditionally.*
> *To chant is to serve.*
> *To meditate is to serve.*

To serve is to make others happier and healthier.
I will serve unconditionally to create a Love Peace Harmony
    Universal Family.
Thank you. Thank you. Thank you.

Heal the Spiritual Body

Now let us practice with The Source Ling Guang Calligraphy *Da Guang Ming* to heal the spiritual body.

A human being has countless souls. A human being has a body soul, souls of all systems, souls of all organs, souls of all cells, cell units, DNA, RNA, spaces between the cells, tiny matter inside the cells, and more.

Souls reincarnate lifetime after lifetime. Souls carry the wisdom, knowledge, and life experience memories of all lifetimes. Souls also carry the blockages of all lifetimes. Applying The Source Ling Guang Calligraphy *Da Guang Ming* for healing the spiritual body is the key for healing all sickness.

Soul is the boss. The importance of healing the spiritual body cannot be explained enough by words.

Heal and transform the soul first; then healing
and transformation of every aspect of life will follow.

We can also express this sacred key for healing in another way:

Heal and transform the spiritual body first; then healing
and transformation of the mental, emotional,
and physical bodies will follow.

Apply the Four Power Techniques with The Source Ling Guang Calligraphy *Da Guang Ming* to heal the spiritual body:

Body Power. Sit up straight in a chair with your back free and clear. Place one palm on your lower abdomen below the navel. Place your other palm over this palm. Connect with The Source Ling Guang Calligraphy *Da Guang Ming*.

Soul Power. Say *hello*:

> *Dear Divine,*
> *Dear Tao, The Source,*
> *Dear Source Ling Guang Calligraphy* Da Guang Ming,
> *Dear the saints, Heaven's saints' animals, and Heaven, Divine and*
>   *Tao Source treasures connected with The Source Ling Guang*
>   *Calligraphy* Da Guang Ming,
> *I love you, honor you, and appreciate you.*
> *Please heal and transform my spiritual body.*
> *I am very grateful.*
> *Thank you.*

Mind Power. Visualize golden or rainbow light from the calligraphy and from Heaven, Mother Earth, the Divine, Tao, and The Source pouring into your spiritual body, transforming the soul mind body blockages from all lifetimes.

Sound Power. Chant aloud or silently:

> *Da Guang Ming* (pronounced *dah gwahng ming*) *heals and*
>   *transforms my spiritual body. Thank you.*
> *Da Guang Ming heals and transforms my spiritual body. Thank you.*
> *Da Guang Ming heals and transforms my spiritual body. Thank you.*
> *Da Guang Ming heals and transforms my spiritual body. Thank you.*
> *Da Guang Ming heals and transforms my spiritual body. Thank you.*
> *Da Guang Ming heals and transforms my spiritual body. Thank you.*
> *Da Guang Ming heals and transforms my spiritual body. Thank*
>   *you . . .*

Please stop reading now to practice for ten minutes. The longer you practice per time, and the more often you practice, the better.

Gratitude and Forgiveness Practice

> *Dear Divine,*
> *Dear Tao, The Source,*

Dear The Source Ling Guang Calligraphy Da Guang Ming,

Dear all of the saints, Heaven's saints' animals, and Heaven's treasures within The Source Ling Guang Calligraphy Da Guang Ming,

I am extremely honored to receive your blessing to remove my spiritual blockages in order to heal my spiritual body.

Please forgive my ancestors and me for all of the mistakes that we have made in all lifetimes.

I deeply apologize for all of our mistakes.

I will serve others unconditionally to make others happier and healthier.

I will work together with humanity and all souls to create a Love Peace Harmony Universal Family.

Thank you. Thank you. Thank you.

The Source Ling Guang Calligraphy *San Jiao Chang Tong— The Pathway of Qi and Body Fluid Flows Freely*

You have learned in chapter 1 that San Jiao (*three areas*, pronounced *sahn jee-yow*) is the pathway of qi and body fluid. Qi is yang. Body fluid is yin. Body fluid includes blood, urine, saliva, and liquids of the organs and cells. In traditional Chinese medicine there is a renowned statement:

Qi xing xue xing, qi zhi xue ning

"Qi" means *energy*. "Xing" means *move*. "Xue" means *blood*. "Zhi" means *sluggish*. "Ning" means *stagnant*. "Qi xing xue xing, qi zhi xue ning" (pronounced *chee shing shooeh shing, chee jr shooeh ning*) means *if qi moves, blood moves; if qi is sluggish, blood is stagnant.*

Traditional Chinese medicine applies three major modalities to treat sickness:

1. Chinese herbs
2. Acupuncture and moxibustion
3. Chinese massage (*tui na*)

To move qi and blood is the key for all three methods of treatment in traditional Chinese medicine. San Jiao is the most important pathway of qi and body fluid in the whole body.

"San Jiao" means *three spaces inside the body.* They are the *Upper Jiao, Middle Jiao, and Lower Jiao.* San Jiao (pronounced *sahn jee-yow*) is the pathway of qi and body fluid. The Upper Jiao is the area above the diaphragm, and includes the heart, lungs, and brain. The Middle Jiao is the area between the diaphragm and the level of the navel, and includes the gallbladder, stomach, and spleen. The Lower Jiao is the area between the level of the navel and the genital area, and includes the kidneys, urinary bladder, liver, small and large intestines, and reproductive and sexual organs.

Another renowned statement of traditional Chinese medicine is:

San Jiao chang tong, bai bing xiao chu

"Chang tong" (pronounced *chahng tawng*) means *flows freely.* "Bai" (pronounced *bye*) means *hundreds.* In Chinese "hundreds" represents *all.* "Bing" means *sickness.* "Xiao chu" (pronounced *shee-yow choo*) means *removed.*

"San Jiao chang tong, bai bing xiao chu" (pronounced *sahn jee-yow chahng tawng, bye bing shee-yow choo*) means *if the most important pathway of qi and body fluid flows freely, all sickness disappears.*

The Source Ling Guang Calligraphy *San Jiao Chang Tong* is The Source Field, which carries the jing qi shen of The Source. It also is the message. I emphasize again the relationship among jing qi shen:

Shen directs qi. Qi directs jing.

Shen is soul, spirit, information, or message. Qi is vital energy. Jing is matter. When you give the message, qi follows. When qi flows, blood follows.

San Jiao Chang Tong is one of the most important messages for healing all sickness. San Jiao is the pathway of qi and body fluid. When you chant *San Jiao Chang Tong*, the message promotes the free flow of qi and body fluid. When qi and body fluid flow freely, all sicknesses will receive healing. Therefore, The Source Ling Guang Calligraphy *San Jiao Chang Tong* has power and benefits beyond words.

Apply The Source Ling Guang Calligraphy *San Jiao Chang Tong* with the Four Power Techniques to heal the whole body:

Heal the Whole Body

Body Power. Sit up straight in a chair with your back free and clear. Refer to the color insert near the end of this chapter. Connect with figure 24, The Source Ling Guang Calligraphy *San Jiao Chang Tong.*

Soul Power. Say *hello*:

> *Dear Divine,*
> *Dear Tao, The Source,*
> *Dear all of the saints, Heaven's saints' animals, and Heaven, Divine,*
>   *and Tao Source treasures connected to and carried within The*
>   *Source Ling Guang Calligraphy* San Jiao Chang Tong,
> *I love you, honor you, and appreciate you.*
> *Please heal and transform my whole body.*
> *Thank you.*

Mind Power. Visualize golden and rainbow light from The Source Ling Guang Calligraphy *San Jiao Chang Tong* shining and radiating throughout your whole body, from head to toe, skin to bone.

Sound Power. Chant silently or aloud:

> *Golden and rainbow light from The Source Ling Guang Calligraphy*
>   San Jiao Chang Tong *(pronounced sahn jee-yow chahng tawng)*
>   *heal my whole body. Thank you.*
> *San Jiao Chang Tong, Bai Bing Xiao Chu (pronounced sahn jee-yow*
>   *chahng tawng, bye bing shee-yow choo)*
> *San Jiao Chang Tong, Bai Bing Xiao Chu*
> *San Jiao Chang Tong, Bai Bing Xiao Chu*
> *San Jiao Chang Tong, Bai Bing Xiao Chu*
> *San Jiao Chang Tong, Bai Bing Xiao Chu*

San Jiao Chang Tong, Bai Bing Xiao Chu
San Jiao Chang Tong, Bai Bing Xiao Chu

Golden Light, Rainbow Light
Golden Light, Rainbow Light
Golden Light, Rainbow Light
Golden Light, Rainbow Light
Golden Light, Rainbow Light
Golden Light, Rainbow Light
Golden Light, Rainbow Light . . .

Please stop reading now to practice for ten minutes.

The Source Ling Guang Calligraphy *San Jiao Chang Tong* can be applied for healing any part of the body. Spend more time to practice. There is no time limit. I repeat again: If you have a chronic or life-threatening condition, chant for two hours or more per day. The longer you chant and the more often you chant, the better the results you could receive. Add all of your practice time together to total at least two hours per day.

Come back to this calligraphy often. Anytime you need healing, come back to this calligraphy directly.

Now let us once again do the gratitude and forgiveness practice:

Dear Divine,
Dear Tao, The Source,
Dear The Source Ling Guang Calligraphy San Jiao Chang Tong,
Dear all of the saints, Heaven's saints' animals, and Heaven's
    treasures within The Source Ling Guang Calligraphy San Jiao
    Chang Tong,
I am extremely honored to receive your blessing to heal my body from
    head to toe, skin to bone.
Please forgive my ancestors and me for all of the mistakes that we
    have made in all lifetimes.
Dear all of the people and all the souls that my ancestors and I have
    harmed, hurt, and taken advantage of in the physical body in all
    lifetimes,

I deeply apologize for all of the mistakes we have made.
Please forgive me.
I will serve others unconditionally to make others happier and
  healthier.
I will work with humanity and all souls together to create a Love
  Peace Harmony Universal Family.
Thank you. Thank you. Thank you.

In summary, this is the first time that I have created The Source Ling Guang Calligraphies for healing the spiritual, mental, emotional, and physical bodies. The Source Field within each of the calligraphies has power beyond words, comprehension, and imagination. If you do not receive healing results right away, be patient and confident. Trust and practice more.

There is no limitation to asking for healing by applying The Source Ling Guang Calligraphies. It is vital to practice more and more. After each practice session, please remember to show your respect and gratitude to Heaven by doing the gratitude and forgiveness practice. It will accelerate your healing so that you can receive your own soul healing miracle faster.

The Source Ling Guang Calligraphy is an unconditional universal servant for humanity and all souls.

Practice. Practice. Practice.
Receive more benefits from it.
Create your own soul healing miracles.
Transform every aspect of your life.
Thank you, Divine.
Thank you, Tao, The Source.
Thank you, all The Source Ling Guang Calligraphies.
Thank you, all saints, all saints' animals, all treasures of Heaven, the
  Divine, Tao, and The Source connected to and carried within the
  calligraphies.

Thank you, all kinds of visible and invisible light carried within the calligraphies.

We are extremely honored.

Words are not enough to express our greatest gratitude.

Comprehension is not enough to express our greatest gratitude.

Imagination is not enough to express our greatest gratitude.

Love you. Love you. Love you.

Thank you. Thank you. Thank you.

Conclusion

I AM EXTREMELY HONORED to have been chosen as a servant of humanity and all souls as well as a divine servant, vehicle, and channel in July 2003.

I immediately started to offer Divine Karma Cleansing and Divine Soul Mind Body Transplants. In 2008 Tao (Source) chose me as a servant, vehicle, and channel of Tao to offer Tao Karma Cleansing and Tao Soul Mind Body Transplants.

Since 2003 I have offered thousands of Divine and Tao Karma Cleansings and countless Soul Mind Body Transplants. Divine and Tao service has created hundreds of thousands of soul healing miracles.

The Divine and Tao guided me to create ten books in the Soul Power Series. Now the Divine and Tao have guided me to create the Soul Healing Miracle Series. This is the first book in the series.

The message of the Soul Healing Miracles Series is:

I have the power to create soul healing miracles
to transform all of my life.

You have the power to create soul healing miracles
to transform all of your life.

Together we have the power to create soul healing miracles
to transform all life of humanity and all souls in Mother Earth
and countless planets, stars, galaxies, and universes.

The most important awareness you should have after reading this book is that *you can create your own soul healing miracles.* Some of my Worldwide Representatives have created hundreds of soul healing miracles. My advanced students have also created many soul healing miracles. If you practice dedicatedly with the soul healing techniques and priceless permanent treasures offered in this book, including the Source Ling Guang Calligraphies, you could create soul healing miracles beyond your comprehension.

How can you create soul healing miracles?

I am delighted to summarize the keys to creating your own soul healing miracles:

- Self-clear karma. This is *the* key to create soul healing miracles and to transform every aspect of life, including health, emotions, relationships, finances, and more. *Karma is the root cause of success and failure in every aspect of life.*
- Do Forgiveness Practice regularly. This is the sacred way to self-clear karma.
- Invoke The Source Ling Guang Calligraphies. This is to invoke The Source Sacred Field to remove soul mind body blockages in order to create soul healing miracles to transform all life.
- Receive the permanent Source treasures transmitted through the book. This is one of the greatest honors one could have in all lifetimes.
- Apply the permanent Source treasures you receive through the book. The Source frequency and vibration of these treasures can create soul healing miracles to transform all life.
- Chant the new Source mantras *Tao Guang Zha Shan*, *Hei Heng Hong Ha*, and *Guang Liang Hao Mei*. These mantras can create soul healing miracles because they carry The Source abilities to transform every aspect of all life, including relationships, finances, business, intelligence, and more.
- Practice The Source Ming Men Jin Dan Meditation. This is a powerful new sacred meditation from The Source for healing, rejuvenation, and prolonging life.
- Apply the five-thousand-year-old wisdom and knowledge of traditional Chinese medicine. These are shared in the soul

healing techniques in this book to heal the physical and emotional bodies of the Five Elements.

- Use the Four Power Techniques (Body Power, Soul Power, Mind Power, Sound Power) and the Five Power Techniques (add Breath Power). These are key techniques for every practice to self-heal and to heal others. Using all power techniques together is extremely powerful.
- Open, develop, purify, and promote the flow of the divine energy circle. This is one of the most important and powerful ways to heal all sickness in the spiritual, mental, emotional, and physical bodies.
- Open, develop, purify, and promote the flow of the divine matter circle. This is one of the most important and powerful ways to rejuvenate soul, heart, mind, and body and to prolong life.
- and more

I would like to emphasize again to *do the practices and exercises in this book*. Do them again and again with persistence, sincerity, trust, and more. You could experience a soul healing miracle very quickly. But remember, even after experiencing a soul healing miracle, continue to practice to maintain good health.

Five thousand years ago *The Yellow Emperor's Internal Classic*, the authority book of traditional Chinese medicine, emphasized prevention of sickness as a priority for health. Practice in order to prevent sickness. If we can prevent sickness, why not do it?

Some people could take more time to experience a soul healing miracle. The reason is that some people have very heavy soul mind body blockages. These blockages could have brought chronic or life-threatening conditions for years. It could take time to remove all of the blockages.

There is an ancient statement:

De bing ru shan dao, qu bing ru chou si

"De" means *get*. "Bing" means *sickness*. "Ru" means *just like*. "Shan" means *mountain*. "Dao" means to *collapse*. "Qu" means *remove*. "Chou si" means *spin silk*. "De bing ru shan dao, qu bing ru chou si" (pronounced *duh bing roo shahn dow, chü bing roo cho sz)* means *sickness occurs just like a mountain collapsing; removing sickness is just like spinning silk.*

This ancient statement tells us that sickness can come suddenly and could be very serious, like a mountain falling, but removing sickness could be a slow process, like spinning silk.

If you receive soul healing miracles quickly, congratulations! Continue to practice to maintain your good health.

If you receive a little improvement after receiving the permanent treasures and blessings from the book and practicing, congratulations! Practice more in order to receive soul healing miracles.

If you feel nothing has worked for you, do not think you cannot be healed or that soul healing does not work. You could have very heavy soul mind body blockages related to your condition. It could take time to heal. Do not lose hope. Be patient. Be confident. Trust that you can be healed. Chronic and life-threatening conditions can take time to heal, but miracle healings could happen at any moment. It is vital to practice persistently and show gratitude to the Divine, Tao, and The Source. Your soul healing miracle could be on the way. I wish for you to receive great healing results as soon as possible.

In the ten books of my Soul Power Series I have released, explained, and emphasized one sentence that carries the most profound sacred wisdom and practices:

> **Heal and transform the soul first; then healing**
> **and transformation of the mind and body will follow.**

This sacred wisdom is to explain the process of healing.
Now I am releasing a major new secret.

> **A person's soul gets sick first; then sickness**
> **of the mind and body will follow.**

This sacred wisdom explains the process of becoming sick.

I explained above that when a person gets sick it is just like a mountain collapsing. It could happen quickly and seriously. Many people do not realize that sickness does not happen suddenly. It happens at the soul level first. The soul could be sick for years, and then suddenly sickness manifests at the physical level.

For those who do not experience great results right away, if you understand this secret, you will be patient because your sickness could have been present at the soul level for many years. The soul could have been very sick before the physical sickness appeared. It could take time to heal the soul to restore your health.

Practice. Practice. Practice.

Why have divine servants, vehicles, and channels and Divine Soul Healers created hundreds of thousands of soul healing miracles so quickly? It is because the Divine and Tao have healed the soul of the sickness.

In the last ten years, I have created hundreds of thousands of soul healing miracles, but not all sicknesses can be healed. I emphasize again: if a sickness cannot be healed, the soul mind body blockages of the sickness could be very heavy, especially the soul blockages, which are negative karma.

Even though soul healing miracles may not happen for some very serious conditions, do not lose hope. Trust. Be confident. Believe that the Divine, Tao, and Heaven can help you. Practice persistently. Practice more and more. I wish for you to have good results as soon as possible.

Hundreds of thousands of soul healing miracles have already happened. I am so honored and grateful to the Divine, Tao, and The Source. I am honored to be a servant of humanity and all souls. Visit www. drsha.com, www.youtube.com/zhigangsha, and www.facebook.com/ drandmastersha to read and view many heart-touching and moving soul healing miracle stories that will inspire you to continue to practice in order to create your own soul healing miracles.

Millions of people suffer from chronic and life-threatening conditions. They suffer from emotional imbalances, including anger, depression, anxiety, grief, sadness, worry, and fear. Mother Earth is suffering from natural disasters, including tsunamis, hurricanes, earthquakes, floods, fires, droughts, and more, and all kinds of other challenges, including environmental, economic, and political challenges, war, and more. The suffering of humanity needs to be removed.

The message of the Soul Healing Miracles Series cannot be emphasized enough.

*I have the power to create soul healing miracles
to transform all of my life.*

*You have the power to create soul healing miracles
to transform all of your life.*

*Together we have the power to create soul healing miracles
to transform all life of humanity and all souls in Mother Earth
and countless planets, stars, galaxies, and universes.*

At this historic time on Mother Earth, the Divine and Tao have guided me to release and emphasize ancient and new sacred wisdom and practices in order to empower humanity to create soul healing miracles to heal their spiritual, mental, emotional, and physical bodies and transform all of their lives.

Study. Study. Study.
Practice. Practice. Practice.
You can create soul healing miracles to transform all of your life.
I love all humanity and all souls.
*I have given my life to serve all humanity and all souls by removing
    the suffering of humanity and all souls and creating a Love Peace
    Harmony Universal Family.*

I love my heart and soul
I love all humanity
Join hearts and souls together
Love, peace and harmony
Love, peace and harmony

Acknowledgments

I THANK FROM THE BOTTOM OF MY HEART the beloved thirty-six saints and the Divine, Tao, and The Source Committees who flowed this book through me. All of my books are their books. They are above my head and I flow the entire book from them. I am so honored to be a servant of all of them, humanity, and all souls. I am eternally grateful.

I thank from the bottom of my heart beloved Divine who chose me as a servant of humanity and the Divine to offer Divine Karma Cleansing and all kinds of Soul Mind Body Transplants in July 2003.

The Divine teaches me daily. I have learned directly so much sacred wisdom, knowledge, and practical techniques from the Divine. I am eternally grateful.

I thank from the bottom of my heart beloved Tao (Source), who chose me as a servant of Tao to offer Tao Karma Cleansing and all kinds of Tao Soul Mind Body Transplants.

Tao teaches me sacred wisdom, knowledge, and practical techniques all of the time. I cannot honor Tao enough.

I thank from the bottom of my heart my beloved spiritual fathers and mothers, including Dr. and Master Zhi Chen Guo. Dr. and Master Zhi Chen Guo is the founder of Body Space Medicine and Zhi Neng Medicine. He was one of the most powerful spiritual leaders, teachers, and healers in the world. He taught me the sacred wisdom, knowledge, and practical techniques of soul, mind, and body. I cannot honor and thank him enough.

I thank from the bottom of my heart Professor Liu Da Jun, the world *I Ching* and feng shui authority at Shandong University in China. He taught me profound secrets of *I Ching* and feng shui. I cannot thank him enough. I cannot thank him enough for writing an introduction to this book. I am deeply honored.

I thank from the bottom of my heart Dr. and Professor Liu De Hua. He is a medical doctor and a former university professor in China. He is the 372nd lineage holder of the Chinese "Long Life Star" Peng Zu, the teacher of Lao Zi, the author of *Dao De Jing*. He taught me the secrets, wisdom, knowledge, and practical techniques of longevity. I cannot thank him enough.

I thank from the bottom of my heart Professor Li Qiu Yun. She is a professor of the root law of simplified cursive Chinese calligraphy. She is more than one hundred years old. I am extremely honored to learn from her and to have been able to write the Ling Guang Calligraphies in this book with one stroke per character.

I thank from the bottom of my heart my beloved sacred masters and teachers who wish to remain anonymous. They have taught me sacred wisdom of Xiu Lian. They are extremely humble and powerful. They have taught me priceless secrets, wisdom, knowledge, and practical techniques but they do not want any recognition. I cannot thank them enough.

I thank from the bottom of my heart the saints in Heaven who give Heaven's sacred books through soul communication to me. I cannot appreciate and honor them enough.

I thank from the bottom of my heart my physical father and mother and all of my ancestors. I cannot honor my physical father and mother enough. Their love, care, compassion, purity, generosity, kindness, integrity, confidence, and much more have influenced and touched my heart and soul forever. I cannot thank them enough.

I thank from the bottom of my heart my literary agent, Bill Gladstone. His love, dedication, and professionalism to his clients have touched me deeply. I cannot thank him enough.

I thank Michael Bernard Beckwith for writing the Foreword for the Soul Healing Miracles Series. His service to humanity has touched millions worldwide. I deeply appreciate him and cannot thank him enough.

I thank from the bottom of my heart, Glenn Yeffeth, publisher (BenBella Books) of my Soul Healing Miracle Series. His full support of this new series has touched my heart deeply. I cannot thank him enough.

I thank from the bottom of my heart the publishing team of Jennifer Canzoneri, Monica Lowry, Sarah Dombrowsky, Adrienne Lang, Ty Nowicki, Cathy Lewis, and others for their great support. I cannot thank them enough.

I thank from the bottom of my heart Sylvia Chen, CEO of Universal Soul Service Corp. She has given me unconditional support since 1992. Her invaluable contribution, dedication, and leadership to the mission have deeply touched and moved my heart. As she is also a great philanthropist, I have learned a lot from her about humanitarian service to communities throughout the world. I am deeply grateful and cannot thank her enough.

I thank from the bottom of my heart the business leaders of the mission: Sylvia Chen, Alexandre Gheysen, Master Sabine Parlow, Master Mirva Inkeri, and Master Ximena Gavino; and the soul leaders of the mission: Master Maya Mackie, Master Cynthia Marie Deveraux, Master Francisco Quintero, Master Allan Chuck, Master Peter Hudoba, Master David Lusch, and Master Marilyn Smith, for their unconditional service and great contribution to the mission. I cannot thank them enough.

I thank from the bottom of my heart the marketing team for this book, including Rick Frishman, Master Ximena Gavino, Darcie Rowan, Mary Agnes Antonopolous, Chandra Stewart, and Firuzan Mistry, for their great contribution to the mission. I cannot thank them enough.

I thank from the bottom of my heart my chief editor, Master Allan Chuck, for his excellent editing of this book and all of my other books. He is one of my Worldwide Representatives and a Divine Channel. He has contributed greatly to the mission and his unconditional universal service is one of the greatest examples for all. I cannot thank him enough.

I thank from the bottom of my heart my senior editor, Master Elaine Ward, for her excellent editing of this book and my other books. She is also one of my Worldwide Representatives and a Divine Channel. I thank her deeply for her great contribution to the mission. I cannot thank her enough.

I thank from the bottom of my heart Master Lynda Chaplin, one of my Worldwide Representatives and a Divine Channel. She has designed the figures for this book and my other books, as well as proofread this book. I am extremely grateful. I cannot thank her enough.

I thank from the bottom of my heart Henderson Ong, the Art Director of our mission. His selfless service and great contribution to this book and many other contributions to the mission have deeply touched my heart. I cannot thank him enough.

I thank from the bottom of my heart Rick Riecker and Gloria Kovacevich for their unconditional universal service in proofreading this book. I cannot thank them enough.

I thank from the bottom of my heart Min Lei and Shi Gao for assisting with the Chinese characters and pinyin in this book and my other books. I am very grateful. I cannot thank them enough.

I thank from the bottom of my heart Master Shu-Chin Hsu, one of my Worldwide Representatives and a Divine Channel, and Hui-Ling Lin for their great translation of Professor Liu Da Jun's introduction. I cannot thank them enough.

I thank Master Francisco Quintero, Master Maya Mackie, Master David Lusch, and Master Marilyn Smith, who are my Worldwide Representatives and Divine Channels, for flowing the Divine and Tao soul guidance for the cover design of the book. I cannot thank them enough.

I thank from the bottom of my heart my assistant, Master Cynthia Marie Deveraux, one of my Worldwide Representatives and a Divine Channel. She has typed the whole book and many of my other books. She also offered great insight during the flowing of this book. She has made a great contribution to the mission. I cannot thank her enough.

I thank from the bottom of my heart all of my Worldwide Representatives, Master Maya Mackie, Master Cynthia Marie Deveraux, Master Francisco Quintero, Master Allan Chuck, Master Peter Hudoba, Master David Lusch, Master Sabine Parlow, Master Mirva Inkeri, Master Ximena Gavino, Master Sher O'Rourke, Master Lynne Nusyna, Master Petra Herz, Master Pam Uyeunten, Master Peggy Werner, Master Lynda Chaplin, Master Marilyn Smith, Master Patricia Smith, Master Roger Givens, Master Elaine Ward, Master Elisabeth Koch, Master Maria Sunukjian, Master Trevor Allen, Master Ellen Logan, Master Kirsten Ernst, Master Robyn Rice, Master Shunya Barton, Master Robert Feda, Master Bill Thomas, Master Zoetha Amritam, Master Diane Fujio, Master Prince Gulati, and Master Thai-Siew

Liang. They are servants of humanity and servants, vehicles, and channels of the Divine. They have made incredible contributions to the mission. I thank them all deeply. I cannot thank them enough.

I thank from the bottom of my heart all of my business team leaders and members for their great contribution and unconditional service to the mission. I am deeply grateful. I cannot thank them enough.

I thank from the bottom of my heart the four thousand Divine Healing Hands Soul Healers worldwide for their great healing service to humanity and all souls. I am deeply touched and moved. They have responded to the divine calling to serve. I deeply thank them all.

I thank from the bottom of my heart the Divine Soul Teachers and Healers, Divine Master Teachers, and Soul Operation Master Healers worldwide for their great contribution to the mission. I am deeply touched and moved. I cannot thank them enough.

I thank from the bottom of my heart all of my students and friends worldwide for their unconditional service to humanity. I cannot thank them enough.

I thank from the bottom of my heart my family, including my parents, my wife, her parents, our children, as well as our brothers and sisters. They have all loved and supported me unconditionally. I cannot thank them enough.

May this book serve humanity and Mother Earth to pass through this difficult time in this historic period.

May this book serve humanity to create soul healing miracles to heal, rejuvenate, purify, and transform all life.

May this book bring love, peace, and harmony to humanity, Mother Earth, and all souls in countless planets, stars, galaxies, and universes.

May this book serve your soul journey and the soul journey of humanity.

I am extremely honored to be a servant of you, humanity, and all souls.

I love my heart and soul
I love all humanity
Join hearts and souls together
Love, peace and harmony
Love, peace and harmony

A Special Gift

I am delighted to include three gifts for you and every reader. You can easily access them on my website, www.DrSha.com. Click on the link for the *Soul Healing Miracles* book, or scan the code on the next the page using your smartphone or other device to access the page.

Gift #1. A documentary film, "Soul Healing Miracles with Dr. and Master Sha." Watch the documentary again and again to receive its blessing from The Source frequency and vibration.

Gift #2. Introduction to The Source Ling Guang Calligraphy. Listen to or download an mp3 audio file where I share sacred wisdom and knowledge about the Ling Guang Calligraphies in this book.

Gift #3. Attend two Soul Healing Miracles events as my guest. Every reader may attend two Soul Healing Miracles events of your choice (in person, by teleconference, or via webcast) as my guest. One event would be with me. The other event would be with any of my Worldwide Representatives and Divine Channels. You will receive tremendous blessings for your physical life and soul journey by participating in these events.

I welcome you to join our Love Peace Harmony Universal Family to spread love, peace, harmony, healing, and upliftment to humanity and all souls, and to receive continual blessings as you offer this service.

I have the power to create soul healing miracles
to transform all of my life.

You have the power to create soul healing miracles
to transform all of your life.

Together we have the power to create soul healing miracles
to transform all life of humanity and all souls in Mother Earth
and countless planets, stars, galaxies, and universes.

Open your heart and soul to receive these gifts from The Source and my heart. It is my honor to serve you.

Index

Books of the Soul Power Series

Soul Wisdom: Practical Soul Treasures to Transform Your Life (revised trade paperback edition) Heaven's Library/Atria, 2008. Also available as an audiobook.

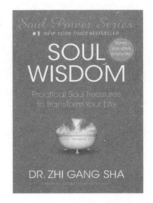

The first book of the Soul Power Series is an important foundation for the entire series. It teaches five of the most important practical soul treasures: Soul Language, Soul Song, Soul Tapping, Soul Movement, and Soul Dance.

Soul Language empowers you to communicate with the Soul World, including your own soul, all spiritual fathers and mothers, souls of nature, and more, to access direct guidance.

Soul Song empowers you to sing your own Soul Song, the song of your Soul Language. Soul Song carries soul frequency and vibration for soul healing, soul rejuvenation, soul prolongation of life, and soul transformation of every aspect of life.

Soul Tapping empowers you to do advanced soul healing for yourself and others effectively and quickly.

Soul Movement empowers you to learn ancient secret wisdom and practices to rejuvenate your soul, mind, and body and prolong life.

Soul Dance empowers you to balance your soul, mind, and body for healing, rejuvenation, and prolonging life.

This book offers two permanent Divine Soul Transplants as gifts to every reader. Includes bonus Soul Song for Healing and Rejuvenation of Brain and Spinal Column MP3 download.

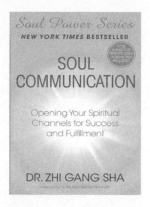

Soul Communication: Opening Your Spiritual Channels for Success and Fulfillment (revised trade paperback edition). Heaven's Library/ Atria, 2008. Also available as an audiobook.

The second book in the Soul Power Series empowers you to open four major spiritual channels: Soul Language Channel, Direct Soul Communication Channel, Third Eye Channel, and Direct Knowing Channel.

The Soul Language Channel empowers you to apply Soul Language to communicate with the Soul World, including your own soul, all kinds of spiritual fathers and mothers, nature, and the Divine. Then, receive teaching, healing, rejuvenation, and prolongation of life from the Soul World.

The Direct Soul Communication Channel empowers you to converse directly with the Divine and the entire Soul World. Receive guidance for every aspect of life directly from the Divine.

The Third Eye Channel empowers you to receive guidance and teaching through spiritual images. It teaches you how to develop the Third Eye and key principles for interpreting Third Eye images.

The Direct Knowing Channel empowers you to gain the highest spiritual abilities. If your heart melds with the Divine's heart or your soul melds with the Divine's soul completely, you do not need to ask for spiritual guidance. You know the truth because your heart and soul are in complete alignment with the Divine.

This book also offers two permanent Divine Soul Transplants as gifts to every reader. Includes bonus Soul Song for Weight Loss MP3 download.

The Power of Soul: The Way to Heal, Rejuvenate, Transform, and Enlighten All Life. Heaven's Library/Atria, 2009. Also available as an audiobook and a trade paperback.

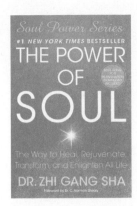

The third book of the Soul Power Series is the flagship of the entire series.

The Power of Soul empowers you to understand, develop, and apply the power of soul for healing, prevention of sickness, rejuvenation, transformation of every aspect of life (including relationships and finances), and soul enlightenment. It also empowers you to develop soul wisdom and soul intelligence, and to apply Soul Orders for healing and transformation of every aspect of life.

This book teaches Divine Soul Downloads (specifically, Divine Soul Transplants) for the first time in history. A Divine Soul Transplant is the divine way to heal, rejuvenate, and transform every aspect of a human being's life and the life of all universes.

This book offers eleven permanent Divine Soul Transplants as a gift to every reader. Includes bonus Soul Song for Rejuvenation MP3 download.

Divine Soul Songs: Sacred Practical Treasures to Heal, Rejuvenate, and Transform You, Humanity, Mother Earth, and All Universes. Heaven's Library/Atria, 2009. Also available as an audiobook and a trade paperback.

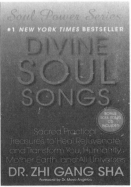

The fourth book in the Soul Power Series empowers you to apply Divine Soul Songs for healing, rejuvenation, and transformation of every aspect of life, including relationships and finances.

Divine Soul Songs carry divine frequency and vibration, with divine love, forgiveness, compassion, and light, that can transform the frequency and vibration of all aspects of life.

This book offers nineteen Divine Soul Transplants as gifts to every reader. Includes bonus Soul Songs CD with seven samples of the Divine Soul Songs that are the main subjects of this book.

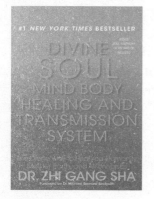

Divine Soul Mind Body Healing and Transmission System: The Divine Way to Heal You, Humanity, Mother Earth, and All Universes. Heaven's Library/Atria, 2009. Also available as an audiobook and a trade paperback.

The fifth book in the Soul Power Series empowers you to receive Divine Soul Mind Body Transplants and to apply Divine Soul Mind Body Transplants to heal and transform soul, mind, and body.

Divine Soul Mind Body Transplants carry divine love, forgiveness, compassion, and light. Divine love melts all blockages and transforms all life. Divine forgiveness brings inner peace and inner joy. Divine compassion boosts energy, stamina, vitality, and immunity. Divine light heals, rejuvenates, and transforms every aspect of life, including relationships and finances.

This book offers forty-six permanent divine treasures, including Divine Soul Transplants, Divine Mind Transplants, and Divine Body Transplants, as a gift to every reader. Includes bonus Soul Symphony of Yin Yang excerpt (MP3 download).

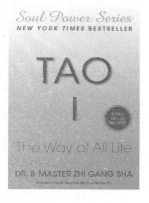

Tao I: The Way of All Life. Heaven's Library/Atria, 2010. Also available as an audiobook.

The sixth book of the Soul Power Series shares the essence of ancient Tao teaching and reveals the Tao Jing, a new "Tao Classic" for the twenty-first century. These new divine teachings reveal how Tao is in every aspect of life, from waking to sleeping to eating and more. This book shares advanced soul wisdom and practical approaches for *reaching* Tao. The new sacred teaching in this book is extremely simple, practical, and profound.

Studying and practicing Tao has great benefits, including the ability to heal yourself and others, as well as humanity, Mother Earth, and all universes; return from old age to the health and purity of a baby; prolong life; and more.

This book offers thirty permanent Divine Soul Mind Body Transplants as gifts to every reader and a fifteen-track CD with Master Sha singing the entire Tao Jing and many other major practice mantras.

Divine Transformation: The Divine Way to Self-clear Karma to Transform Your Health, Relationships, Finances, and More. Heaven's Library/Atria, 2010. Also available as an audiobook.

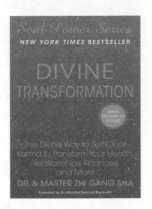

The teachings and practical techniques of this seventh book of the Soul Power Series focus on karma and forgiveness. Bad karma is the root cause of any and every major blockage or challenge that you, humanity, and Mother Earth face. True healing is to clear your bad karma, which is to repay or be forgiven your spiritual debts to the souls you or your ancestors have hurt or harmed in all your lifetimes. Forgiveness is a golden key to true healing. Divine self-clearing of bad karma applies divine forgiveness to heal and transform every aspect of your life.

Clear you karma to transform your soul first; then transformation of every aspect of your life will follow.

This book offers thirty rainbow frequency Divine Soul Mind Body Transplants as gifts to every reader and includes four audio tracks of major Divine Soul Songs and practice chants.

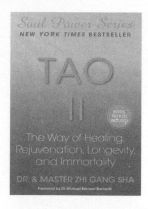

Tao II: The Way of Healing, Rejuvenation, Longevity, and Immortality. Heaven's Library/ Atria, 2010. Also available as an audiobook.

The eighth book of the Soul Power Series is the successor to *Tao I: The Way of All Life. Tao II* reveals the highest secrets and most powerful practical techniques for the Tao journey, which includes one's physical journey and one's spiritual journey.

Tao II gives you the sacred keys for your whole life's practice and shares the Immortal Tao Classic, two hundred and twenty sacred phrases that include not only profound sacred wisdom but also additional simple and practical techniques. *Tao II* explains how to reach *fan lao huan tong*, which means to *transform old age to the health and purity of the baby state*; to prolong life; and to reach immortality to be a better servant for humanity, Mother Earth, and all universes.

This book offers twenty-one Tao Soul Mind Body Transplants as gifts to every reader and includes two audio tracks of major Tao chants for healing, rejuvenation, longevity, and immortality.

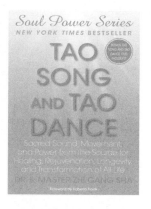

Tao Song and Tao Dance: Sacred Sound, Movement, and Power from the Source for Healing, Rejuvenation, Longevity, and Transformation of All Life. Heaven's Library/ Atria, 2011. Also available as an audiobook.

The ninth book in the Soul Power Series and the third of the Tao series, *Tao Song and Tao Dance* introduces you to the highest and most profound Soul Song. Sacred Tao Song mantras and Tao Dance carry Tao love, which melts all blockages; Tao forgiveness, which brings inner joy and inner peace; Tao compassion, which boosts energy, stamina, vitality, and immunity; and Tao light, which heals, prevents sickness, purifies and rejuvenates soul, heart, mind, and body, and transforms relationships, finances, and every aspect of life.

Includes access to video recording of Master Sha practicing Tao Song mantras for healing, rejuvenation, longevity, and purification.

Divine Healing Hands: Experience Divine Power to Heal You, Animals, and Nature, and Transform All Life. Heaven's Library/Atria, 2012. Also available as an audiobook.

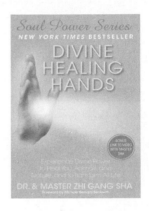

Divine Healing Hands are the Divine's soul light healing hands. They carry divine healing power to heal and to transform relationships and finances. Master Sha has asked the Divine to download Divine Healing Hands to every copy of this tenth book of the Soul Power Series. Every reader of *Divine Healing Hands* will then be able to experience the amazing power of Divine Healing Hands directly twenty times. For the first time, the Divine is giving his Divine Healing Hands to the masses. To receive Divine Healing Hands is to serve humanity and the planet in these critical times. Learn how you can answer the Divine's calling and receive Divine Healing Hands.